D0764909

QUALITATIVE RESEARCH
IN HEALTH CARE

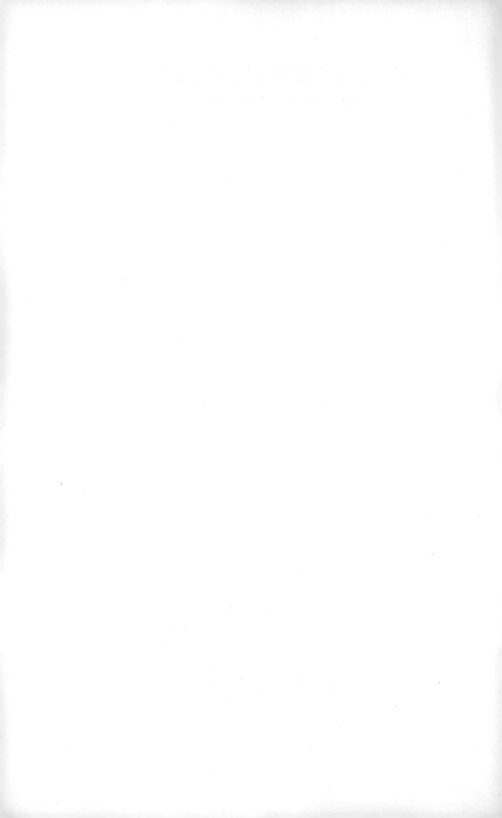

QUALITATIVE RESEARCH IN HEALTH CARE

Edited by

NICHOLAS MAYS

Director of Health Services Research,
King's Fund Policy Institute, London

and

CATHERINE POPE

Lecturer in Social and Behavioural Medicine,
Department of Epidemiology and Public Health,
University of Leicester, Leicester

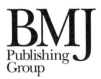

BMJ
Publishing
Group

© BMJ Publishing Group 1996
Second impression 1997

First published in 1996
by the BMJ Publishing Group, BMA House, Tavistock Square,
London WC1H 9JR

British Library Cataloguing in Publication Data

A catalogue record for this book is available from the British Library
ISBN 0–7279–1013–2

Typeset by Apek Typesetters Ltd, Nailsea, Bristol
Printed and bound in Great Britain by Latimer Trend & Company Ltd, Plymouth

Contents

Preface

This book was probably conceived during a conference paper we gave at the Society for Social Medicine Annual Scientific Meeting in September 1991. An edited version of the paper, "Opening the black box," was subsequently published in the *BMJ* and is reproduced at the end of this book. This was a somewhat quirky, theatrical presentation of a fictional dialogue between a director of a health services research unit and a junior sociologist, discussing the tensions between qualitative and quantitative methods.

This dialogue owed much to conversations with colleagues, experiences of working in health and health care research, and our various encounters with clinicians, research funding bodies, and journal editors. The paper was a deliberately provocative depiction of the qualitative–quantitative divide, but behind it lay our conviction that the full range of methods available in health services research should be used as and when the research questions demanded it.

The response to the paper suggested that more information was needed about the methods we had alluded to and the *BMJ* asked us to put together a series of papers looking in detail at a range of methods. In attempting to convey the essence of a wide range of qualitative approaches we drew on the expertise of other researchers involved in health services research. This process culminated in a series of seven papers published in the *BMJ* and collected here.

Chapter 1 sets out the merits of qualitative approaches and indicates where they can be particularly illuminating. Chapter 2 considers the extent to which qualitative methods can lay claim to producing valid results and how researchers might improve the rigour of qualitative work. Each of the subsequent chapters is devoted to one of the principal methods.

The working brief for the series was to outline non-quantitative methods for health care workers and researchers. As a result some of the approaches mentioned may not, strictly, be considered qualitative. For example, many consensus methods generate numerical scores, but their basis is the elicitation of subjective judgments. These methods are used increasingly widely in medical settings, yet misunderstood. What all the methods described here have in common, however, is their divergence from more quantitative, experimental, and statistical models of research with which clinicians and other health researchers may be more familiar.

This book could not pretend to give a definitive description of all qualitative methods. Thus, for example, we have not been able to look at other forms of research, which frequently employ qualitative methods, such as action research, which is being used increasingly in health care settings,[1] nor have we included documentary methods,[2 3] which have been employed in the study of health related issues such as tranquilliser dependency.[4]

Secondly, we have not explicitly examined the epistemological and methodological debates which surround the use of qualitative as opposed to quantitative methods in the social sciences. We do not look at the theoretical and philosophical underpinnings of different methods and the important tensions and conflicts between the different social science perspectives.[5 6 7]

Rather, we simply indicate that different methods enable the researcher to gain access to different types of knowledge. These types of knowledge are not necessarily hierarchically arranged, nor can they be added together to provide a bigger or better picture of what is "really" happening. They may even yield conflicting perspectives. We suggest that qualitative and quantitative methods can be viewed as complementary and be used to generate a richness of understanding and interpretation.

The aim of this book, then, is to serve as a practical guide for doctors, nurses, and other researchers otherwise unfamiliar with qualitative methods, to outline what these methods consist of, how they might be carried out, and the common pitfalls and the benefits of each. Care has been taken to provide examples of the application of each method to the study of health and health care. The references in each chapter and further reading lists provide helpful pointers to more detailed reading.

In putting together this volume we wish to thank many colleagues and friends, in particular the authors of the chapters, who have encouraged and inspired us. We are also grateful to the editorial team at the *BMJ* for their willingness to take qualitative

research seriously and for their enthusiasm in seeing the series into
book form.

Catherine Pope
Nicholas Mays
October 1995

1 Hart E, Bond M. *Action research for health and social care: a guide to practice.* Milton Keynes:
Open University Press, 1995.
2 Plummer K. *Documents of life: an introduction to problems and literature of a humanistic method.*
London: Allen and Unwin, 1983.
3 Scott J. *A matter of record.* Cambridge: Polity Press, 1990.
4 Gabe J, Gustafsson U, Bury M. Mediating illness: newspaper coverage of transquilliser
dependence. *Soc Hlth Illness* 1991;13:332–53.
5 Bryman A. *Quantity and quality in social research.* London: Unwin Hyman, 1988.
6 Bryman A. The debate about quantitative and qualitative research: a question of method or
epistemology? *Br J Sociology* 1984;35(1):75–92.
7 Hammersley M. Deconstructing the qualitative–quantitative divide. In: Brannen J. *Mixing
methods: qualitative and quantitative research.* Aldershot: Avebury, 1992:39–55.

1 Qualitative methods in health and health services research

CATHERINE POPE, NICK MAYS

Qualitative research methods have a long history in the social sciences and deserve to be an essential component in health and health services research. Qualitative and quantitative approaches to research tend to be portrayed as antithetical; the aim of this book is to show the value of a range of qualitative techniques and how they can complement quantitative research.

Aims of this book

Medical advances, increasing specialisation, rising patient expectations, and the sheer size and diversity of health service provision mean that today's health professionals work in an increasingly complex arena. The wide range of research questions generated by this complexity has encouraged the search for new ways of conducting research. The rapid expansion of research on and about health and health services, and the relatively recent demarcation of a distinct field of "health services research" depend heavily on doctors and other health professionals being investigators, participants, and peer reviewers. Yet some of the most important questions in health services concern the organisation and culture of those who provide health care, such as why the findings of randomised controlled trials are often difficult to apply in day to day clinical practice. The social science methods appropriate to studying such phenomena are very different from the methods familiar to many health professionals.

1

Although the more qualitative approaches found in certain of the social sciences may seem alien alongside the experimental, quantitative methods used in clinical and biomedical research, they should be an essential component of health services research—not just because they enable us to access areas not amenable to quantitative research, such as lay and professional health beliefs, but also because qualitative description is a prerequisite of good quantitative research, particularly in areas that have received little previous investigation. A good example of this is the study of the social consequences of the application of new genetic techniques to screening for genetic disease.[1] New genetic technologies place individuals, couples, and families in novel circumstances facing unprecedented decisions about such things as reproduction, transmission of genetic defects, and the response to information about predisposition to particular diseases. The starting point for social research in this field is therefore an attempt to understand how and why people conceptualise genetic risks and why they behave as they do when faced with them.

The aim of this book is to introduce some of the main qualitative research methods currently used in health care research and to indicate how they can be appropriately and fruitfully employed. The chapters review observation, in depth interviews, focus groups, consensus methods, and case studies, all of which doctors and other health professionals are increasingly coming into contact with. We hope that by making clear what these methods entail, how they are used, and how they can be evaluated, they will seem less strange and be viewed as valuable tools in the methodological tool box of health and health services research. Chapters 3 to 6 concentrate on specific qualitative methods, while Chapter 2 deals with validity and reliability in qualitative research. Box 1 provides short definitions of some of the terms used in qualitative research which appear in the rest of the book.

Although relatively uncommon in health services research, qualitative methods have long been used in the social sciences. Social anthropology, for example, was founded on studies in which an understanding of the customs and behaviour of people from remote lands was gathered by researchers who spent time living in those societies, often learning their languages so they could participate while observing. In a similar way, these naturalistic methods—in essence, watching, joining in, talking, and reading about the group being studied—are used by qualitative sociologists

Box 1—Glossary of terms used in the series

Epistemology—theory of knowledge; scientific study which deals with the nature and validity of knowledge

Naturalistic research—non-experimental research in naturally occurring settings

Social anthropology—social scientific study of peoples, cultures, and societies; particularly associated with the study of traditional cultures

Induction—process of moving from observations/data towards generalisations, hypotheses, or theory; **grounded theory**—hypothesising inductively from data, notably using subjects' own categories, concepts, etc; opposite of **deduction**, process of data gathering to test predefined theory or hypotheses

Purposive or systematic sampling—deliberate choice of respondents, subjects, or settings, as opposed to **statistical sampling**, concerned with the representativeness of a sample in relation to a total population. **Theoretical sampling** links this to previously developed hypotheses or theories

Fieldnotes—collective term for records of observation, talk, interview transcripts, or documentary sources. Typically includes a field diary which provides a record of the chronological events and development of research as well as the researcher's own reactions to, feeling about, and opinions of the research process

Content analysis—systematic examination of text (field notes) by identifying and grouping themes and coding, classifying, and developing categories.

Constant comparison—iterative method of content analysis where each category is searched for in the entire data set and all instances are compared until no new categories can be identified. **Analytic induction**—use of constant comparison specifically in developing hypotheses, which are then tested in further data collection and analysis

Triangulation—use of three or more different research methods in combination; principally used as a check of validity

Observation—systematic watching of behaviour and talk in naturally occurring settings. **Participant observation**—observation in which the researcher also occupies a role or part in the setting in addition to observing

In depth interviews—face to face conservation with the purpose of exploring issues or topics in detail. Does not use pre-set questions, but is shaped by a defined set of topics or issues

Focus groups—method of group interview which explicitly includes and uses the group interaction to generate data

Consensus methods include **Delphi** and **nominal group techniques** and **consensus development conferences.** They provide a way of synthesising information and dealing with conflicting evidence, with the aim of determining extent of agreement within a selected group

Case studies focus on one or a limited number of settings; used to explore contemporary phenomenon, especially where complex interrelated issues are involved. Can be exploratory, explanatory, or descriptive or a combination of these

Validity—extent to which a measurement truly reflects the phenomenon under scrutiny

Hawthorne effect—impact of the researcher on the research subjects or setting, notably in changing their behaviour

Reliability—extent to which a measurement yields the same answer each time it is used

Box 2—The overstated dichotomy between quantitative and qualitative social science

	Qualitative	Quantitative
Social theory:	Action	Structure
Methods:	Observation, interview	Experiment, survey
Question:	What is X? (classification)	How many Xs? (enumeration)
Reasoning:	Inductive	Deductive
Sampling method:	Theoretical	Statistical
Strength:	Validity	Reliability

to study the familiar: our own society. Health care is just one area where these techniques have been applied to study subjects such as the organisation of health services, interactions between doctors and patients, and the changing roles of the health professions.

What are qualitative methods?

The common feature of the methods discussed in this book is that they do not primarily seek to provide quantified answers to research questions. So what exactly do they aim to do? The goal of qualitative research is the development of concepts which help us to understand social phenomena in natural (rather than experimental) settings, giving due emphasis to the meanings, experiences, and views of all the participants. As a result they are particularly suited, for example, to understanding how it is that health education messages on stopping smoking can be well known to teenagers or young working class women but not perceived as relevant to their everyday lives.[23] Qualitative studies are concerned with answering questions such as "What is X and how does X vary in different circumstances, and why?" rather than "How many Xs are there?" Since qualitative research does not generally seek to enumerate, it is viewed as the antithesis of the quantitative method; indeed, the two approaches are frequently presented as adversaries in a methodological battle. This view is often reinforced by highlighting a corresponding split in social theory between theories concerned with delineating social structure and those interested in understanding social action or meaning. Box 2 presents a caricature of the differences between qualitative and quantitative methods in the social sciences which are often marshalled as evidence of the essential incompatibility of the two approaches.

The randomised controlled trial, with its focus on hypothesis testing through experiment controlled by means of randomisation, can be seen as the epitome of the quantitative method. Answering the "what is X" question, though, is the foundation of quantification: until something is classified it cannot be measured. Moreover, because health care deals with people and people are, on the whole, more complex than the subjects of the natural sciences, there is a whole set of questions about human interaction, and how people interpret interaction, which health professionals may need answers to. Experimental and quantitative methods are less well suited to answer these questions.

Consider an example from research on diabetes. There can be no doubt that quantitative methods, including randomised controlled trials, have contributed to advances in the treatment of this disease.[4] As well as knowing that glycaemic control is effective in reducing long term complications, health professionals may need answers to additional questions—for example, those concerned with patient behaviour. For a general practitioner, knowing that intensive insulin therapy works may be secondary to knowing whether the patient will comply with the treatment. This is where qualitative research can be useful. Indeed, there is a body of work which examines and explains why patients do not comply with treatment regimens.[5]

The rigid demarcation of qualitative and quantitative research as opposing traditions that is shown in box 2 does not encourage movement or interaction between the two camps. In effect, researchers on either side become entrenched and are often ignorant of each other's work. Within sociology there is a growing recognition that the quantitative-qualitative distinction has created an unnecessary divide, and this has done little to assist the progress of the discipline.[6] In health services research the differences between qualitative and quantitative methods continue to be overstated and misunderstood.[7]

The dichotomy described in box 2 suggests that whereas quantitative methods aim for reliability (that is, consistency on retesting) through the use of tools such as standardised questionnaires, qualitative methods score more highly on validity, by getting at how people really behave and what people actually mean when they describe their experiences, attitudes, and behaviours. In addition, the reasoning implicit in qualitative work is held to be inductive (moving from observation to hypothesis) rather than hypothesis testing or deductive. For example, much methodological writing in the qualitative tradition emphasises that in order to get behind respondents' formal public statements and behaviour to uncover their personal perceptions and actual day to day actions, it is important not to impose *a priori* categories and concepts from the researcher's own professional knowledge on to the process of data collection. Rather than starting with a research question or a hypothesis that precedes any data collection, the researcher is encouraged not to separate the stages of design, data collection, and analysis, but to go backwards and forwards between the raw data and the process of conceptualisation, thereby making sense of the data throughout the period of data collection.[8]

In the methodological debate, these distinctions are frequently presented as clear cut, but the contrasts are more apparent than real. In health services research, because of its applied nature, much research is driven, not by the theoretical stance of the researcher, but by a specific practical problem which is turned into a research question. As Brannen notes, "There is no necessary or one to one correspondence between epistemology and methods."[9] As she suggests, the choice of method and how it is used can perfectly well be matched to what is being studied rather than to the disciplinary or methodological leanings of the researcher. It is therefore possible to envisage deductive pieces of qualitative research.

How can qualitative methods complement quantitative ones?

It would seem more fruitful for the relation between qualitative and quantitative methods to be characterised as complementary rather than exclusive. There are at least three ways in which this can be achieved. Firstly, as noted above, qualitative work can be conducted as an essential preliminary to quantitative research. Qualitative techniques such as observation, in depth interviews, and focus groups (which are covered in subsequent papers in this series) can be used to provide a description and understanding of a situation or behaviour. At their most basic, these techniques can be used simply to discover the most comprehensible terms or words to use in a subsequent survey questionnaire. An excellent recent example of this was the qualitative research conducted to establish which sexual terms would be most appropriate to use in the British national survey of sexual attitudes and lifestyles.[10] This work highlighted several ambiguities and misunderstandings. "The meaning of many terms–'vaginal sex', 'oral sex', 'penetrative sex', 'heterosexual'—was unclear to a sizeable enough number of people to threaten substantially the overall validity of response."

The second way qualitative methods can be used is to supplement quantitative work. This can be part of the validation process, as in "triangulation,"[11] where three or more methods are used and the results compared for convergence (for example, a large scale survey, focus groups, and a period of observation), or as part of a multimethod approach which examines a particular phenomenon or topic on several different levels.[9] This is not simply a matter of joining two techniques, or tacking one on the end of a project. Researchers need to be aware of the different types of answers derived from different methods. Cornwell's work looking at the health of families in the East end of London was able to distinguish powerfully between the public and private accounts provided by respondents.[12] Though a survey may pick up the public account, a series of in depth interviews are needed to get at the private, often contradictory and complex beliefs people hold. This theme is pursued by Britten in Chapter 4. It would be invidious to suggest that one or the other source was the more valid; suffice it to say that different research settings and different methods allow access to different levels of knowledge. None the less, combining methods can help to build a wider picture, and this is especially productive when used to explore the findings of previous research, such as the observational examination of the surgical decision making process by Bloor *et al*, which built on an epidemiological study of the widespread variations in the rates of common surgical procedures (box 3).[13]

The third way in which qualitative research can complement quantitative work is by exploring complex phenomena or areas not amenable to quantitative research. The value of this sort of stand alone qualitative research is increasingly widely recognised in studies of health service organisation and policy.[14] It may be especially useful in looking at health services in times of reform or policy change from the point of view of the patients, professionals, and managers affected. In Chapter 7, Keen and Packwood provide

---

Box 3—Two stage investigation of the association between differences in geographic incidence of operations on the tonsils and adenoids and local differences in specialists' clinical practices[13]

I Epidemiological study—documenting variations

Analysis of 12 months' routine data on referral, acceptance, and operation rates for new patients under 15 years in two Scottish regions known to have significantly different 10 year operation rates for tonsils and adenoids.

Found significant differences between similar areas within regions in referral, acceptance, and operation rates that were not explained by disease incidence

Operation rates influenced, in order of importance, by:

- Differences between specialists in propensity to list for operations
- Differences between GPs in propensity to refer
- Differences between areas in symptomatic mix of referrals.

II Sociological study—explaining how and why variations come about

Observation of assessment routines undertaken in outpatient departments by six consultants in each region on a total of 493 under 15s.

Found considerable variation between specialists in their assessment practices (search procedures and decision rules), which led to differences in disposals, which in turn created local variations in surgical incidence.

"High operators" tended to view a broad spectrum of clinical signs as important and tended to assert the importance of examination findings over the child's history; "low operators" gave the examination less weight in deciding on disposal and tended to judge a narrower range of clinical features as indicating the need to operate.

---

one example of how qualitative methods can be used to examine the consequences of changes in resource allocation and management practices at the micro level within NHS hospitals. In addition, qualitative work can reach aspects of complex behaviours, attitudes, and interactions which quantitative methods cannot. As a result it has been extremely useful for examining clinical decision making by probing and exploring both the declared and the implicit or tacit routines and rules which doctors use.[15 16]

In this book the aim is to show how qualitative methods can, and do, enrich our knowledge of health and health care. It is not that qualitative methods are somehow superior to quantitative ones—such a position merely perpetuates the quantitative-qualitative dichotomy—but that we need a range of methods at our fingertips if we are to understand the complexities of modern health care. "What is involved is not a crossroads where we have to go left or right. A better analogy is a complex maze where we are repeatedly faced with decisions, and where paths wind back on one another. The prevalence of the distinction between qualitative and quantitative method tends to obscure the complexity of the problems that face us and threatens to render our decisions less effective than they might otherwise be."[17]

Further reading

Patton MQ. *Qualitative evaluation and research methods.* London: Sage, 1990.
Bryman, A. *Quality and quantity in social research.* London: Unwin Hyman, 1988.

1 Mitchie S, McDonald V, Marteau T. Understanding responses to predictive genetic testing: a ground theory approach. *Psychology and Health* (in press).
2 Amos A, Currie C, Hunt SM. The dynamnics and processes of behavioural change in five classes of health related behaviour: findings from qualitative research. *Health Education Research 1991;* 6:443–53.
3 Graham H. *When life's a drag: women smoking and disadvantage.* London: HMSO, 1993.
4 Diabetes Control and Complications. Trial Research Group. The effect of intensive treatment of diabetes on the development of long-term complications in insulin-dependent diabetes mellitus. *N Engl J Med* 1993;**329**:977–86.
5 Morgan M, Watkins C. Managing hypertension: beliefs and responses to medication among cultural groups. *Sociology of Health and Illness* 1988;**10**:561–78.
6 Abell P. Methodological achievements in sociology over the past few decades with special reference to the interplay of qualitative and quantitative methods. In: Bryant C, Becker H, eds. *What has sociology achieved.* London: Macmillan, 1990:94–116.
7 Pope, C, Mays N. Opening the black box: an encounter in the corridors of health services research. *BMJ* 1993;**306**:315–18.
8 Bryman A, Burgess R, eds. *Analysing qualitative data.* London: Routledge, 1993.
9 Brannen J, ed. *Mixing methods: qualitative and quantitative research.* Aldershot: Avebury, 1992:3–38.
10 Wellings K, Field J, Johnson A, Wadsworth J. *Sexual behaviour in Britain: the national survey of sexual attitudes and lifestyles.* Harmondsworth: Penguin 1994.
11 Denzin N. *The research act.* London: Butterworth, 1970.
12 Cornwell J. *Hard earned lives.* London: Tavistock, 1984.
13 Bloor MJ, Venters GA, Samphier ML. Geographical variation in the incidence of operations on the tonsils and adenoids: an epidemiological and sociological investigation. *J Laryngol Otol* 1976;**92**:791–801, 883–95.
14 Pollitt C, Harrison S, Hunter DJ, Marnoch G. No hiding place: on the discomforts of researching the contemporary policy process. *Journal of Social Policy* 1990;**19**:169–90.
15 Silverman D. *Communication and medical practice.* London: Sage, 1987.
16 Strong P. *The ceremonial order of the clinic.* London: Routledge, 1979.
17 Hammersley M. Deconstructing the qualitative-quantitative divide. In: Brannen J, ed. *Mixing methods: qualitative and quantitative research.* Aldershot: Avebury, 1992:39–55.

2 Rigour and qualitative research

NICHOLAS MAYS, CATHERINE POPE

Various strategies are available within qualitative research to protect against bias and enhance the reliability of findings. This chapter gives examples of the principal approaches and summarises them into a methodological checklist to help readers of reports of qualitative projects to assess the quality of the research.

Criticisms of qualitative research

In the health field—with its strong tradition of biomedical research using conventional, quantitative, and often experimental methods—qualitative research is often criticised for lacking scientific rigour. To label an approach "unscientific" is peculiarly damning in an era when scientific knowledge is generally regarded as the highest form of knowing. The most commonly heard criticisms are, firstly, that qualitative research is merely an assembly of anecdote and personal impressions, strongly subject to researcher bias; secondly, it is argued that qualitative research lacks reproducibility—the research is so personal to the researcher that there is no guarantee that a different researcher would not come to radically different conclusions; and, finally, qualitative research is criticised for lacking generalisability. It is said that qualitative methods tend to generate large amounts of detailed information about a small number of settings.

Is qualitative research different?

The pervasive assumption underlying all these criticisms is that quantitative and qualitative approaches are fundamentally different in their ability to ensure the validity and reliability of their findings. This distinction, however, is more one of degree than of type. The problem of the relation of a piece of research to some presumed underlying "truth" applies to the conduct of any form of social research. "One of the greatest methodological fallacies of the last half century in social research is the belief that science is a particular set of techniques; it is, rather, a state of mind, or attitude, and the organisational conditions which allow that attitude to be expressed."[1] In quantitative data analysis it is possible to generate statistical representations of phenomena which may or may not be fully justified since, just as in qualitative work, they will depend on the judgment and skill of the researcher and the appropriateness to the question answered of the data collected. All research is selective—there is no way that the researcher can in any sense capture the literal truth of events. All research depends on collecting particular sorts of evidence through the prism of particular methods, each of which has its strengths and weaknesses. For example, in a sample survey it is difficult for the researcher to ensure that the questions, categories, and language used in the questionnaire are shared uniformly by respondents and that the replies returned have the same meanings for all respondents. Similarly, research that relies exclusively on observation by a single researcher is limited by definition to the perceptions and introspection of the investigator and by the possibility that the presence of the observer may, in some way that is hard to characterise, have influenced the behaviour and speech that was witnessed. Britten and Fisher summarise the position neatly by pointing out that "there is some truth in the quip that quantitative methods are reliable but not valid and that qualitative methods are valid but not reliable."[2]

Strategies to ensure rigour in qualitative research

As in quantitative research, the basic strategy to ensure rigour in qualitative research is systematic and self conscious research design, data collection, interpretation, and communication. Beyond this, there are two goals that qualitative researchers should seek to achieve: to create an account of method and data which can stand independently so that another trained researcher could analyse the same data in the same way and come to essentially the same conclusions; and to produce a plausible and coherent

11

explanation of the phenomenon under scrutiny. Unfortunately, many qualitative researchers have neglected to give adequate descriptions in their research reports of their assumptions and methods, particularly with regard to data analysis. This has contributed to some of the criticisms of bias from quantitative researchers.

Yet the integrity of qualitative projects can be protected throughout the research process. The remainder of this chapter discusses how qualitative researchers attend to issues of validity, reliability, and generalisability.

Sampling

Much social science is concerned with classifying different "types" of behaviour and distinguishing the "typical" from the "atypical". In quantitative research this concern with similarity and difference leads to the use of statistical sampling so as to maximise external validity or generalisability. Although statistical sampling methods such as random sampling are relatively uncommon in qualitative investigations, there is no reason in principle why they cannot be used to provide the raw material for a comparative analysis, particularly when the researcher has no compelling *a priori* reason for a purposive approach. For example, a random sample of practices could be studied in an investigation of how and why teamwork in primary health care is more and less successful in different practices. However, since qualitative data collection is generally more time consuming and expensive than, for example, a quantitative survey, it is not usually practicable to use a probability sample. Furthermore, statistical representativeness is not a prime requirement when the objective is to understand social processes.

An alternative approach, often found in qualitative research and often misunderstood in medical circles, is to use systematic, non-probabilistic sampling. The purpose is not to establish a random or representative sample drawn from a population but rather to identify specific groups of people who either possess characteristics or live in circumstances relevant to the social phenomenon being studied. Informants are identified because they will enable exploration of a particular aspect of behaviour relevant to the research. This approach to sampling allows the researcher deliberately to include a wide range of types of informants and also to select key informants with access to important sources of knowledge.

"Theoretical" sampling is a specific type of non-probability sampling in which the objective of developing theory or explanation guides the process of sampling and data collection.[3] Thus, the analyst makes an initial selection of informants; collects, codes, and analyses the data; and produces a preliminary theoretical explanation before deciding which further data to collect and from whom. Once these data are analysed, refinements are made to the theory, which may in turn guide further sampling and data collection. The relation between sampling and explanation is iterative and theoretically led.

To return to the example of the study of primary care team working, some of the theoretically relevant characteristics of general practices affecting variations in team working might be the range of professions represented in the team, the frequency of opportunities for communication among team members, the local organisation of services, and whether the practice is in an urban, city, or rural area. These factors could be identified from other similar research and within existing social science theories of effective and ineffective team working and would then be used explicitly as sampling categories. Though not statistically representative of general practices, such a sample is theoretically informed and relevant to the research questions. It also minimises the possible bias arising from selecting a sample on the basis of convenience.

Ensuring the reliability of an analysis

In many forms of qualitative research the raw data are collected in a relatively unstructured form such as tape recordings or transcripts of conversations. The main ways in which qualitative researchers ensure the retest reliability of their analyses is in maintaining meticulous records of interviews and observations and by documenting the process of analysis in detail. While it is possible to analyse such data singlehandedly and use ways of classifying and categorising the data which emerge from the analysis and remain implicit, more explicit group approaches, which perhaps have more in common with the quantitative social sciences, are increasingly used. The interpretative procedures are often decided on before the analysis. Thus, for example, computer software is available to facilitate the analysis of the content of interview transcripts.[4] A coding frame can be developed to characterise each utterance (for example, in relation to the age, sex, and role of the speaker; the

13

topic; and so on), and transcripts can then be coded by more than one researcher.[5] One of the advantages of audiotaping or video-taping is the opportunity the tapes offer for subsequent analysis by independent observers.

The reliability of the analysis of qualitative data can be enhanced by organising an independent assessment of transcripts by additional skilled qualitative researchers and comparing agreement between the raters. For example, in a study of clinical encounters between cardiologists and their patients which looked at the differential value each derived from the information provided by echocardiography, transcripts of the clinic interviews were analysed for content and structure by the principal researcher and by an independent panel, and the level of agreement was assessed.[6]

Safeguarding validity

Alongside issues of reliability, qualitative researchers give attention to the validity of their findings. "Triangulation" refers to an approach to data collection in which evidence is deliberately sought from a wide range of different, independent sources and often by different means (for instance, comparing oral testimony with written records). This approach was used to good effect in a qualitative study of the effects of the introduction of general management into the NHS. The accounts of doctors, managers, and patient advocates were explored in order to identify patterns of convergence between data sources to see whether power relations had shifted appreciably in favour of professional managers and against the medical profession.[7]

Validation strategies sometimes used in qualitative research are to feed the findings back to the participants to see if they regard the findings as a reasonable account of their experience[8] and to use interviews or focus groups with the same people so that their reactions to the evolving analysis become part of the emerging research data.[9] If used in isolation these techniques assume that fidelity to the participants' commonsense perceptions is the touchstone of validity. In practice, this sort of validation has to be set alongside other evidence of the plausibility of the research account since different groups are likely to have different perspectives on what is happening.[10]

A related analytical and presentational issue is concerned with the thoroughness with which the researcher examines "negative" or "deviant" cases—those in which the researcher's explanatory scheme appears weak or is contradicted by the evidence. The researcher should give a fair account of these occasions and try to explain why the data vary.[11] In the same way, if the findings of a single case study diverge from those predicted by a previously stated theory, they can be useful in revising the existing theory in order to increase its reliability and validity.

Validity and explanation

It is apparent in qualitative research, particularly in observational studies (see Chapter 3 for more on observational methods), that the researcher can be regarded as a research instrument.[12] Allowing for the inescapable fact that purely objective observation is not possible in social science, how can the reader judge the credibility of the observer's account? One solution is to ask a set of questions: how well does this analysis explain why people behave in the way they do; how comprehensible would this explanation be to a thoughtful participant in the setting; and how well does the explanation it advances cohere with what we already know?

This is a challenging enough test, but the ideal test of a qualitative analysis, particularly one based on observation, is that the account it generates should allow another person to learn the "rules" and language sufficiently well to be able to function in the research setting. In other words, the report should carry sufficient conviction to enable someone else to have the same experience as the original observer and appreciate the truth of the account.[13] Few readers have the time or inclination to go to such lengths, but this provides an ideal against which the quality of a piece of qualitative work can be judged.

The development of "grounded theory" another response to this problem of objectivity. Under the strictures of grounded theory, the findings must be rendered through a systematic account of a setting that would be clearly recognisable to the people in the setting (by, for example, recording their words, ideas, and actions) while at the same time being more structured and self consciously explanatory than anything that the participants themselves would produce.

Attending to the context

Some pieces of qualitative research consist of a case study carried out in considerable detail in order to produce a naturalistic account of everyday life. For example, a researcher wishing to observe care in an acute hospital around the clock may not be able to study more than one hospital. Again the issue of generalisability, or what can be learnt from a single case, arises. Here, it is essential to take care to describe the context and particulars of the case study and to flag up for the reader the similarities and differences between the case study and other settings of the same type. A related way of making the best use of case studies is to show how the case study contributes to and fits with a body of social theory and other empirical work.[12] Chapter 7 discusses qualitative case studies in more detail.

Collecting data directly

Another defence against the charge that qualitative research is merely impressionistic is that of separating the evidence from secondhand sources and hearsay from the evidence derived from direct observation of behaviour in situ. It is important to ensure that the observer has had adequate time to become thoroughly familiar with the milieu under scrutiny and that the participants have had the time to become accustomed to having the researcher around. It is also worth asking whether the observer has witnessed a wide enough range of activities in the study site to be able to draw conclusions about typical and atypical forms of behaviour—for example, were observations undertaken at different times? The extent to which the observer has succeeded in establishing an intimate understanding of the research setting is often shown in the way in which the subsequent account shows sensitivity to the specifics of language and its meanings in the setting.

Minimising researcher bias in the presentation of results

Although it is not normally appropriate to write up qualitative research in the conventional format of the scientific paper, with a rigid distinction between the results and discussion sections of the account, it is important that the presentation of the research allows the reader as far as possible to distinguish the data, the analytic framework used, and the interpretation.[1] In quantitative research these distinctions are conventionally and neatly presented in the methods section, numerical tables, and the accompanying commentary. Qualitative research depends in much larger part on producing a convincing account.[14] In trying to do this it is all too easy to construct a narrative that relies on the reader's trust in the

16

Form of doctor's questions to parents at a paediatric cardiology clinic[15]

Question	No of times asked
Random sample of children without handicap (n = 22):	
Is he/she well?	11
From your point of view, is he/she a well baby?	2
Do you notice anything wrong with her/him?	1
From the heart point of view, she/he's active?	1
How is he/she	4
Questions not asked	3
Children with Down's syndrome (n = 12)	
Is he/she well	0
From your point of view, is he/she a well baby?	1
Do you notice anything wrong with her/him?	0
As far as his/her heart is concerned, does he/she get breathless?	1
Does she/he get a few chest infections?	1
How is he/she (this little boy/girl) in himself/herself?	6
Question not asked	3

integrity and fairness of the researcher. The equivalent in quantitative research is to present tables of data setting out the statistical relations between operational definitions of variables without giving any idea of how the phenomena they represent present themselves in naturally occurring settings.[1] The need to quantify can lead to imposing arbitrary categories on complex phenomena, just as data extraction in qualitative research can be used selectively to tell a story that is rhetorically convincing but scientifically incomplete.

The problem with presenting qualitative analyses objectively is the sheer volume of data customarily available and the relatively greater difficulty faced by the researcher in summarising qualitative data. It has been suggested that a full transcript of the raw data should be made available to the reader on microfilm or computer disk,[11] although this would be cumbersome. Another partial solution is to present extensive sequences from the original data (say, of conversations), followed by a detailed commentary.

Another option is to combine a qualitative analysis with some quantitative summary of the results. The quantification is used merely to condense the results to make them easily intelligible; the approach to the analysis remains qualitative since naturally occurring events identified on theoretical grounds are being counted. The table above shows how Silverman compared the format of the doctor's initial questions to parents in a paediatric cardiology clinic when the child was not handicapped with a

17

Questions to ask of a qualitative study

- Overall, did the researcher make explicit in the account the theoretical framework and methods used at every stage of the research?

- Was the context clearly described?

- Was the sampling strategy clearly described and justified?

- Was the sampling strategy theoretically comprehensive to ensure the generalisability of the conceptual analyses (diverse range of individuals and settings, for example)?

- How was the fieldwork undertaken? Was it described in detail?

- Could the evidence (fieldwork notes, interview transcripts, recordings, documentary analysis, etc) be inspected independently by others; if relevant, could the process of transcription be independently inspected?

- Were the procedures for data analysis clearly described and theoretically justified? Did they relate to the original research questions? How were themes and concepts identified from the data?

- Was the analysis repeated by more than one researcher to ensure reliability?

- Did the investigator make use of quantitative evidence to test qualitative conclusions where appropriate?

- Did the investigator give evidence of seeking out observations that might have contradicted or modified the analysis?

- Was sufficient of the original evidence presented systematically in the written account to satisfy the sceptical reader of the relation between the interpretation and the evidence (for example, were quotations numbered and sources given)?

---

smaller number of cases when the child had Down's syndrome. A minimum of interpretation was needed to contrast the two sorts of interview.[15 16]

Assessing a piece of qualitative research

This chapter has shown some of the ways in which researchers working in the qualitative tradition have endeavoured to ensure the rigour of their work. It is hoped that this summary will help the prospective reader of reports of qualitative research to identify some of the key questions to ask when trying to assess its quality. A range of helpful checklists has been published to assist readers of quantitative research assess the design[17] and statistical[18] and economic[19] aspects of individual published papers and review articles.[20] Likewise, the contents of this chapter have been condensed into a checklist for readers of qualitative studies, covering design, data collection, analysis, and reporting (box). We hope that the checklist will give readers of studies in health and health care research that use qualitative methods the confidence to subject them to critical scrutiny.

Further reading

Hammersley M. *Reading ethnographic research*. London: Longman, 1990.

1 Dingall R. 'Don't mind him—he's from Barcelona': qualitative methods in health studies. In: Daly J, MacDonald I, Willis, E. eds. *Researching health care: designs, dilemmas, disciplines*. London: Tavistock/Routledge, 1992: 161–75.
2 Britten N, Fisher B. Qualitative research and general practice [editorial]. *Br J Gen Pract* 1993;43:270–1.
3 Glaser BG, Strauss AL. *The discovery of grounded theory*. Chicago: Aldine, 1967.
4 Seidel J, Clark JA. The ethnograph: a computer program for the analysis of qualitative data. *Qualitative Sociology* 1984;7:110–25.
5 Krippendorff K. *Content analysis: an introduction to its methodology*. London: Sage: 1980.
6 Daly J, MacDonald I, Willis E. Why don't you ask them? A qualitative research framework for investigating the diagnosis of cardiac normality. In: Daly J, MacDonald I, Willis E, eds. *Researching health care: designs, dilemmas, disciplines*. London: Tavistock/Routledge, 1992:189–206.
7 Pollitt C, Harrison S, Hunter DJ, Marnoch G. No hiding place: on the discomforts of researching the contemporary policy process. *Journal of Social Policy* 1990;19:169–90.
8 McKeganey NP, Bloor MJ. On the retrieval of sociological descriptions: respondent validation and the critical case of ethnomethodology. *International Journal of Sociology and Social Policy* 1981;1:58–59.
9 Oakley A. *The sociology of housework*. Oxford: Martin Robertson, 1974.
10 Brannen J. Combining qualitative and quantitative approaches: an overview. In: *Mixing methods: qualitative and quantitative research*. Aldershot: Avebury, 1992:3–37.
11 Waitzkin H. On studying the discourse of medical encounters: a critique of quantitative and qualitative methods and a proposal for reasonable compromise. *Med Care* 1990;28:473–88.
12 Mechanic D. Medical sociology: some tensions among theory, method and substance. *J. Health Soc Behav* 1989;30:147–60.
13 Fielding N. Ethnography. In Gilbert N, ed. *Researching social life*. London: Sage, 1993, 154–71.
14 Silverman D. Telling convincing stories: a plea for cautious positivism in case studies. In: Glassner B, Moreno J, eds. *The qualitative-quantitative distinction in the social sciences*. Dordrecht: Kluwer, 1989:57–77.
15 Silverman D. Applying the qualitative method to clinical care. In: Daly J, MacDonald I, Willis E, eds. *Researching health care: designs, dilemmas, disciplines*. London: Tavistock/Routledge, 1992:176–88.
16 Silverman D. The child as a social object: Down's syndrome children in a paediatric cardiology clinic. *Sociology of Health and Illness* 1981;3:254–74.
17 Fowkes FGR, Fulton PM. Critical appraisal of published research: introductory guidelines. *BMJ* 1991;302:1136–40.
18 Gardner MJ, Machin D, Campbell MJ. Use of check lists in assessing the statistical content of medical studies. *BMJ* 1986;292:810–2.
19 Department of Clinical Epidemiology and Biostatistics. How to read clinical journals. VII. To understand an economic evaluation (part B). *Can Med Assoc J* 1984;130:1542–9.
20 Oxman AD, Guyatt GH. Guidelines for reading literature reviews. *Can Med Assoc J* 1988;138:697–703.

3 Observational methods in health care settings

NICHOLAS MAYS, CATHERINE POPE

Clinicians used to observing individual patients, and epidemiologists trained to observe the course of disease, may be forgiven for misunderstanding the term observational method as used in qualitative research. In contrast to the clinician or epidemiologist, the qualitative researcher systematically watches people and events to find out about behaviours and interactions in natural settings. Observation, in this case, epitomises the idea of the researcher as the research instrument. It involves "going into the field"—describing and analysing what has been seen. In health care settings, this method has been insightful and illuminating, but it is not without pitfalls for the unprepared researcher.

The term "observational methods" seems to be a source of some confusion in medical research circles. Qualitative observational studies are very different from the category of observational studies (non-experimental research designs) used in epidemiology, nor are they like the clinical observation of a patient. Observational methods used in social science involve the systematic, detailed observation of behaviour and talk: watching and recording what people do and say. Goffman neatly captured this distinct research method with his recommendation that, in order to learn about a social group, one should "submit oneself in the company of the members to the daily round of petty contingencies to which they are subject."[1] Thus, observational methods can involve asking

---

Box 1—Observational research roles[2]

Complete participant	Covert observation
Participant as observer	Overt observation—mutual awareness of the research
Observer as participant	Essentially a one shot interview with no enduring relationship based on lengthy observation
Complete observer	Experimental design, no participation

---

questions and analysing documents, but the primary focus on observation makes it distinct from a qualitative research interview (see Chapter 4) or history taking during patient consultation. Another crucial point about qualitative observation is that it takes place in natural settings not experimental ones; hence, this type of work is often described as "naturalistic research."

Research roles

In an attempt to minimise the impact on the environment being studied the researcher sometimes adopts a "participant observer" role, becoming involved in the activities taking place while also observing them. The degree of participation varies according to the nature of the setting and the research questions, but broadly corresponds to the first two research roles described in Gold's typology (box 1).[2] There are obviously important ethical considerations about the decision to conduct covert research, and for this reason examples of this type of observational study are rare. However, its use may be justified in some settings, and it has been used to research sensitive topics such as homosexuality[3] and difficult to access areas such as fascist organisations[4] and football hooliganism.[5] Overt research—Gold's "participant as observer"— may pose fewer ethical dilemmas, but this may be offset by the group or individuals reacting to being observed. At its most basic, having a researcher observing actions may stimulate modifications in behaviour or action—the so-called "Hawthorne effect,"[6] or encourage introspection or self questioning among those being researched. In his classic study of street gangs in the United States, Whyte recounted how a key group member said, "You've slowed me up plenty since you've been down here. Now when I do something I have to think what Bill Whyte would want to know about it and how I can explain it. Before I used to do things by instinct."[7]

In addition to these potential problems for the subjects of observational research, there are important considerations for researchers "entering the field." In essence these involve "getting in and getting out." In the initial phases there may be problems gaining access to a setting, and then in striking up sufficient rapport and empathy with the group to enable research to be conducted. In medical settings, such as a hospital ward, this may involve negotiating with several different staff groups ranging from consultants and junior doctors, to nurse managers, staff nurses, social workers, and auxiliary professions. Once "inside" there is the problem of avoiding "going native"; that is, becoming so immersed in the group culture that the research agenda is lost, or that it becomes extremely difficult or emotionally draining to exit the field and conclude the data collection.

What can observation tell us that other methods cannot?

Given these difficulties, observational methods may seem a peculiar choice for studying health and health services. However, an important advantage of observation is that it can help to overcome the discrepancy between what people say and what they actually do. It circumvents the biases inherent in the accounts people give of their actions caused by factors such as the wish to present themselves in a good light, differences in recall, selectivity, and the influences of the roles they occupy. For these reasons, observational methods are particularly well suited to the study of the working of organisations and how the people within them perform their functions. It may also uncover behaviours or routines of which the participants themselves may be unaware. For example, Jeffery's observation of casualty wards in Edinburgh indicated that, because of the conflicting demands and pressures on staff, some patients, who were seen as inappropriate attenders, were labelled as "normal rubbish" and treated differently from "good" patients, who were viewed as more deserving.[8] A similar picture emerges from Hughes's work on the decisions made by reception clerks when patients present themselves at casualty department.[9] It is unlikely that interviews alone would have elicited these different patterns of care. Indeed the labelling of certain cases as "normal rubbish" may have been so embedded in the culture of the casualty setting that only an outsider or newcomer to the scene would have considered it noteworthy.

Another observational study provides an example of how qualitative work can build on existing quantitative research.[10] Against the background of large variations in rates of common surgical procedures such as hysterectomy, cholecystectomy, and tonsillectomy, Bloor observed ear, nose, and throat outpatient clinics to see how decisions to admit children for surgery were made. He systematically analysed how surgeons made their decisions to operate and discovered that individual doctors had different "rules of thumb" for coming to a decision. While one surgeon might take clinical signs as the chief indication for surgery, another might be prepared to operate in the absence of such indications at the time of consultation if there was evidence that repeated episodes of tonsillitis were severely affecting a child's education. Understanding the behaviour of these surgeons, knowing why they made their decisions, provided considerable insight into how the variation in surgical rates occurred.

Similar variation and patterning occurs in the statistics on inpatient waiting lists: some surgeons have long lists, others do not; some specialties have long waits, others do not. An observational study showed that rules and routines akin to those discovered by Bloor could be discerned in the day to day management of waiting lists.[11] Surgical and administrative preferences were important in deciding who came off the list. Different reasons for admitting a patient might range from case mix demands for teaching juniors, through ensuring a balanced list, to the ease with which a patient could be contacted and offered admission. Thus, observing how waiting lists work can indicate which policy and administrative changes are likely to have an impact in reducing lists and which are not: a policy which assumed that waiting lists operated as first come, first served queues would be unlikely to affect the day to day routines described above.

Some rules about observation

Sampling

Before any recording and analysis can take place, the setting to be observed has to be chosen. As in other qualitative research, this sampling is seldom statistically based. Instead, it is likely to be purposive, whereby the researcher deliberately samples a particular group or setting (see Chapter 2 for more on this). The idea of this type of sampling is not to generalise to the whole population but to indicate common links or categories shared between the setting observed and others like it. At its most powerful, the single case can demonstrate features or provide categories relevant to a wide number of settings. Goffman's observation of mental hospitals in the 1960s generated the valuable concept of the "total institution," of which the asylum was one example alongside others such as prisons and monasteries.[1]

Recording

Qualitative observation involves watching and recording what people say and do. As it is impossible to record everything, this process is inevitably selective and relies heavily on the researcher to act as the research instrument and document the world he or she observes. Therefore it is vital that the observations are systematically recorded and analysed, either through the traditional medium of field notes written during or immediately after the events occur or by using audio or video recording facilities. From his unique position as a patient in a tuberculosis sanatorium, Roth was able to record events as they happened,[13] but such situations are rare and most researchers, whether in covert or more participative roles, find that recording necessitates the development of memory skills and frequent trips to the lavatory to "write up."

The systematic recording of data in qualitative observation distinguishes it from other types of observation such as a tourist recording with a camcorder or a nosey neighbour peering over the fence. Even with video and sound recording it is impossible to "get everything," but as far as possible the researcher aims to record exactly what happened, including his or her own feelings and responses to the situations witnessed. The subjective nature of this type of research contrasts with the objective stance aspired to in the experimental method, but in fact it is a crucial component of the process of analysing qualitative observational data. The researcher usually keeps a field diary or record of the research process to detail events, personal reactions to events, and changes in his or her views over time. Frequently this is the basis of tentative hypotheses or the evolution of systems of classification. In developing classifications or hypotheses it is particularly important to detail any contra-

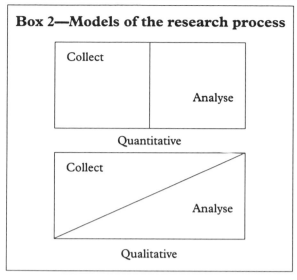

Box 2—Models of the research process

dictory or negative cases—the unusual, out of the ordinary things which often reveal most about the setting or situation. Tentative classifications and the search for negative cases during the data collection are important facets of the analytic technique used in observational research.

Analysis

The fieldnotes gathered during observational research are likely to be detailed, highly descriptive accounts and are therefore cumbersome. As descriptions alone they cannot provide explanations. The researcher's task is to sift and decode the data to make sense of the situation, events, and interactions observed. Often this analytical process starts during the data collection phase, a quite different model of the research process to that found in quantitative research, where data collection is completed before any analysis begins (box 2).

Just as the data are systematically recorded, so they are also systematically analysed. Various ways of dealing with observational data have been described, including "analytic induction" and "constant comparison."[14] Stripped of their theoretical trappings, these methods are all variants of content analysis and involve an iterative process of developing categories from the transcripts or fieldnotes, testing them against hypotheses, and refining them. This analytical process is described in detail by Bloor, based on the

---

Box 3—Analysis

Stages in the analysis of field notes in a qualitative study of ear, nose, and throat surgeons' disposal decisions for children referred for possible tonsillectomy and adenoidectomy (T&A)[11]

(1) Provisional classification—For each surgeon all cases categorised according to the disposal category used (for example, T&A or tonsillectomy alone)

(2) Identification of provisional case features—Common features of cases in each disposal category identified (for example, most T&A cases found to have three main clinical signs present)

(3) Scrutiny of deviant cases—Include in (2) or modify (1) to accommodate deviant cases (for example, T&A performed when only two of three signs present)

(4) Identification of shared case features—Features common to other disposal categories (history of several episodes of tonsillitis, for example)

(5) Derivation of surgeons' decision rules—From the common case features (for example, case history more important than physical examination)

(6) Derivation of surgeons' search procedures (for each decision rule)—The particular clinical signs looked for by each surgeon

Repeat (2) to (6) for each disposal category

---

observational study of ear, nose, and throat clinics described earlier (box 3).[15]

As with quantitative work, it is important that evidence from the data is presented to support the conclusions reached. This can take the form of examples of specific cases, descriptions of events, or quotations. The validity of observational accounts relies on the truthful and systematic representation of the research; in many ways it is honesty which separates the observational account from a novel. Hughes says that observational studies should communicate the culture and rules of the setting well enough to allow another researcher to learn them and "pass" as a member of the group.[16] This is not an easy task, and observational research is therefore particularly demanding of the individual researcher.

This chapter has indicated how observational methods can be used to "reach the parts that other methods cannot." Done well, there is no reason why observation should not be as systematic, rigorous, or valid as other research styles and deserve its place in the health researcher's methodological tool box.

Further reading

Fielding N. *Researching social life*. London: Sage, 1993.
Goffman E. *Asylums*. Harmondsworth: Penguin, 1961.
Strong PM. *The ceremonial order of the clinic*. London: Routledge, 1979.

1 Goffman E. *Asylums*. Harmondsworth: Penguin, 1961.
2 Gold R. Roles in sociological field investigation. *Social Forces* 1958;36:217–23.
3 Humphreys L. *Tearoom trade: impersonal sex in public places*. Chicago: Aldine, 1970.
4 Fielding N. *The National Front*. London: Routledge and Kegan Paul, 1981.
5 Pearson G. *Hooligan: a history of respectable fears*. London: Macmillan, 1983.
6 Roethlisberger FJ, Dickson WJ. *Management and the worker*. Cambridge, MA: Harvard University Press, 1939.
7 Whyte WF. *Street corner society: the social structure of an Italian slum*. Chicago: Chicago University Press, 1955.
8 Jeffery R. Normal rubbish: deviant patients in casualty departments. *Sociology of Health and Illness* 1979;1:90–108.
9 Hughes D. Paper and people: the work of the casualty reception clerk. *Sociology of Health and Illness* 1979;11:382–408.
10 Bloor M. Bishop Berkeley and the adenotonsillectomy enigma: an exploration of the social construction of medical disposals. *Sociology* 1976;10:43–61.
11 Pope C. Trouble in store: some thoughts on the management of waiting lists. *Sociology of Health and Illness* 1991; 13:193–212.
12 Mays N, Pope C. Rigour in qualitative research. *BMJ* 1995;311:109–12.
13 Roth J. *Timetables: structuring the passage of time in hospital treatment and other careers*. New York: Bobbs Merrill, 1963.
14 Bryman A, Burgess R, eds. *Analysing qualitative data*. London: Routledge, 1993.
15 Bloor M. On the analysis of observational data: a discussion of the worth and uses of inductive techniques and respondent validation. *Sociology* 1978;12:545–52.
16 Hughes J. *Sociological analysis: methods of discovery*. London: Nelson, 1976.

4 Qualitative interviews in medical research

NICKY BRITTEN

Much qualitative research is interview based, and this chapter provides an outline of qualitative interview techniques and their application in medical settings. It explains the rationale for these techniques and shows how they can be used to research kinds of questions that are different from those dealt with by quantitative methods. Differing types of qualitative interviews are described, and the way in which they differ from clinical consultations is emphasised. Practical guidance for conducting such interviews is given.

Types of qualitative interview

Practising clinicians routinely interview patients during their clinical work, and they may wonder whether simply talking to people constitutes a legitimate form of research. In sociology and related disciplines, however, interviewing is a well established research technique. There are three main types: structured, semistructured, and in depth interviews (box 1).

Structured interviews consist of administering structured questionnaires, and interviewers are trained to ask questions (mostly fixed choice) in a standardised manner. For example, interviewees might be asked: "Is your health: excellent, good, fair or poor?" Though qualitative interviews are often described as being unstructured in order to contrast them with this type of formalised quantitative interview, the term "unstructured" is misleading as no interview is completely devoid of structure: if it were, there would be no guarantee that the data gathered would be appropriate to the research question.

Box 1—Types of interviews

- Structured
  Usually with a structured questionnaire
- Semistructured
  Open ended questions
- Depth
  One or two issues covered in great detail
  Questions are based on what the interviewee says

Semistructured interviews are conducted on the basis of a loose structure consisting of open ended questions that define the area to be explored, at least initially, and from which the interviewer or interviewee may diverge in order to pursue an idea in more detail. Continuing with the same example, interviewees might initially be asked a series of questions such as: "What do you think good health is?", "How do you consider your own health?", and so on.

Depth interviews are less structured than this, and may cover only one or two issues, but in much greater detail. Such an interview might begin with the interviewer saying, "This research study is about how people think about their own health. Can you tell me about your own health experiences and what you think of your health?" Further questions from the interviewer would be based on what the interviewee said and would consist mostly of clarification and probing for details.

Clinical and qualitative research interviews have very different purposes. Although the doctor may be willing to see the problem from the patient's perspective, the clinical task is to fit that problem into an appropriate medical category in order to choose an appropriate form of management. The constraints of most consultations are such that any open ended questioning needs to be brought to a conclusion by the doctor within a fairly short time. In a qualitative research interview the aim is to discover the interviewee's own framework of meanings and the research task is to avoid imposing the researcher's structures and assumptions as far as possible. The researcher needs to remain open to the possibility that the concepts and variables that emerge may be very different from those that might have been predicted at the outset.

Qualitative interview studies address different questions from those addressed by quantitative research. For example, a quantitative epidemiological approach to the sudden infant death syndrome might measure statistical correlates of national and regional variations in incidence. In a qualitative study Gantley et al interviewed mothers of young babies in different ethnic groups to understand their child rearing practices and hence discover possible factors contributing to the low incidence of sudden infant death in Asian populations.[1] A quantitative study of single-handed general practitioners might compare their prescribing and referral rates, out of hours payments, list sizes, and immunisation and cervical cytology rates with those of general practitioners in partnerships. A recent qualitative study examined the concerns of singlehanded general practitioners during semistructured interviews and identified the problems perceived by this group of doctors.[2] Qualitative research can also open up different areas of research such as hospital consultants' views of their patients[3] or general practitioners' accounts of uncomfortable prescribing decisions.[4]

Conducting interviews

Qualitative interviewers try to be interactive and sensitive to the language and concepts used by the interviewee, and they try to keep the agenda flexible. They aim to go below the surface of the topic being discussed, explore what people say in as much detail as possible, and uncover new areas or ideas that were not anticipated at the outset of the research. It is vital that interviewers check that they have understood respondents' meanings instead of relying on their own assumptions. This is particularly important if there is obvious potential for misunderstanding—for example, when a clinician interviews someone unfamiliar with medical terminology. Clinicians should not assume that interviewees use medical terminology in the same way that they do.

Patton said that good questions in qualitative interviews should be open ended, neutral, sensitive, and clear to the interviewee.[5] He listed six types of questions that can be asked: those based on behaviour or experience, on opinion or value, on feeling, on knowledge, and on sensory experience and those asking about demographic or background details (box 2). It is usually best to start with questions that the interviewee can answer easily and then proceed to more difficult or sensitive topics. Most interviewees are willing to provide the kind of information the researcher wants, but

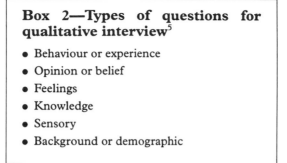

Box 2—Types of questions for qualitative interview[5]

- Behaviour or experience
- Opinion or belief
- Feelings
- Knowledge
- Sensory
- Background or demographic

they need to be given clear guidance about the amount of detail required. It is possible to collect data even in stressful circumstances.[6]

The less structured the interview, the less the questions are determined and standardised before the interview occurs. Most qualitative interviewers will have a list of core questions that define the areas to be covered. Unlike quantitative interviews based on highly structured questionnaires, the order in which questions are asked will vary, as will the questions designed to probe the interviewee's meanings. Wordings cannot be standardised because the interviewer will try to use the person's own vocabulary when framing supplementary questions. Also, during the course of a qualitative study, the interviewer may introduce further questions as he or she becomes more familiar with the topic being discussed.

All qualitative researchers need to consider how they are perceived by interviewees and the effects of characteristics such as class, race, sex, and social distance on the interview. This question becomes more acute if the interviewee knows that the interviewer is also a doctor. An interviewee who is already a patient or likely to become one may wish to please the doctor by giving the responses he or she thinks the doctor wants. It is best not to interview one's own patients for research purposes, but if this cannot be avoided, patients should be given permission to say what they really think, and they should not be corrected if they say things that doctors think are wrong (for example, that antibiotics are a suitable treatment for viral infections).

Interviewers are also likely to be asked questions by interviewees during the course of an interview. The problem with this is that in answering questions, clinical researchers may undo earlier efforts

---

Box 3—Whyte's directiveness scale for analysing interviewing technique[8]

1 Making encouraging noises
2 Reflecting on remarks made by the informant
3 Probing on the last remark by the informant
4 Probing an idea preceding the last remark by the informant
5 Probing an idea expressed earlier in the interview
6 Introducing a new topic
(1 = least directive, 6 = most directive)

---

not to impose their own concepts on the interview. If questions are not answered, this may reduce the interviewee's willingness to answer the interviewer's subsequent questions. One solution is to say that such questions can be answered at the end of the interview, although this is not always a satisfactory response.[7]

Researcher as research instrument

Qualitative interviews require considerable skill on the part of the interviewer. Experienced doctors may feel that they already possess the necessary skills, and indeed many are transferable. To achieve the transition from consultation to research interview, clinical researchers need to monitor their own interviewing technique, critically appraising tape recordings of their interviews and asking others for their comments. The novice research interviewer needs to notice how directive he or she is being, whether leading questions are being asked, whether cues are picked up or ignored, and whether interviewees are given enough time to explain what they mean. Whyte devised a six point directiveness scale to help novice researchers analyse their own interviewing technique (box 3).[8] The point is not that non-directiveness is always best, but that the amount of directiveness should be appropriate. Some informants are more verbose than others, and it is vital that interviewers maintain control of the interview. Patton provided three strategies for maintaining control: knowing the purpose of the interview, asking the right questions to get the information needed, and giving appropriate verbal and non-verbal feedback (box 4).[5]

Some common pitfalls for interviewers that have been identified

---

Box 4—Maintaining control of the interview[5]

- Knowing what it is you want to find out
- Asking the right questions to get the information you need
- Giving appropriate verbal and non-verbal feedback

---

by Field and Morse include outside interruptions, competing distractions, stage fright, awkward questions, jumping from one subject to another, and the temptation to counsel interviewees (box 5).[9] Awareness of these pitfalls can help the interviewer to develop ways of overcoming them.

Recording interviews

There are various ways of recording qualitative interviews: notes written at the time, notes written afterwards, and audiotaping. Writing notes at the time can interfere with the process of interviewing, and notes written afterwards are likely to miss out some details. In certain situations, written notes are preferable to audiotaping, but most people will agree to having an interview tape

---

Box 5—Common pitfalls in interviewing[9]

- Interruptions from outside (telephone, etc)
- Competing distractions (children, etc)
- Stage fright for interviewer or interviewee
- Asking interviewee embarrassing or awkward questions
- Jumping from one subject to another
- Teaching (for example, giving interviewee medical advice)
- Counselling (for example, summarising responses too early)
- Presenting one's own perspective, thus potentially biasing the interview
- Superficial interviews
- Receiving secret information (for example, suicide threats)
- Translators (for example, inaccuracy)

---

recorded, although it may take them a little while to speak freely in front of a machine. It is vitally important to use good quality equipment which has been tested beforehand and with which the interviewer is familiar. Transcription is an immensely time consuming process, as each hour's worth of interview can take six or seven hours to transcribe, depending on the quality of the tape. The costing of any interview based study should include adequate transcription time.

Identifying interviewees

Sampling strategies are determined by the purpose of the research project.[9] Statistical representativeness is not normally sought in qualitative research (see Chapter 3). Similarly, sample sizes are not determined by hard and fast rules, but by other factors such as the depth and duration of the interview and what is feasible for a single interviewer. Large qualitative studies do not often interview more than 50 or 60 people, although there are exceptions.[11] Sociologists conducting research in medical settings often have to negotiate access with great care, although this is unlikely to be a problem for clinicians conducting research in their own place of work. Nevertheless, the researcher still needs to approach the potential interviewee and explain the purpose of the research, emphasising that a refusal will not affect future treatment. An introductory letter should also explain what is involved and the likely duration of the interview and should give assurances about confidentiality. Interviews should always be conducted at interviewees' convenience, which for people who work during the day will often be in the evening. The setting of an interview affects the content, and it is usually preferable to interview people at home.

Conclusion

Qualitative interviewing is a flexible and powerful tool which can open up many new areas for research. It can enable practising clinicians to investigate research questions of immediate relevance to their everyday work, which would otherwise be difficult to investigate. Few researchers would consider embarking on a new research technique without some form of training, and training in research interviewing skills is available from universities and specialist research organisations.

Further reading

Fontana A, Frey JH. Interviewing: the art of science. In: Denzin NK, Lincoln YS, eds. *Handbook of qualitative research*. London: Sage, 1994:361–76.

Mishler EG. *Research interviewing: context and narrative*. Cambridge, MA: Harvard University Press, 1986.

1 Gantley M, Davies DP, Murcott A. Sudden infant death syndrome: links with infant care practices. *BMJ* 1993;**306**:16–20.
2 Green JM. The views of singlehanded general practitioners: a qualitative study. *BMJ* 1993;**307**:607–10.
3 Britten N. Hospital consultants' views of their patients: *Sociology of Health and Illness* 1991;**13**:83–97.
4 Bradley CP. Uncomfortable prescribing decisions: a critical incident study. *BMJ* 1992;**304**:294–6.
5 Patton MQ. *How to use qualitative methods in evaluation*. London: Sage, 1987:108–43.
6 Cannon S. Social research in stressful settings: difficulties for the sociologist studying the treatment of breast cancer. *Sociology of Health and Illness* 1989;**11**:62–77.
7 Oakley A. Interviewing women: a contradiction in terms. In: Roberts H, ed. *Doing feminist research*. London: Routledge and Kegan Paul, 1981:30–61.
8 Whyte WF. Interviewing in field research. In: Burgess RG, ed. *Field research: a sourcebook and field manual*. London: George Allen and Unwin, 1982: 111–22.
9 Field PA, Morse JM. *Nursing research: the application of qualitative approaches*. London: Chapman and Hall, 1989.
10 Mays N, Pope C. Rigour and qualitative research. *BMJ*; 1995;**311**:109–12.
11 Holland J, Ramazanoglu, C. Scott S, Sharpe S, Thomson R. Sex, gender and power: young women's sexuality in the shadow of AIDS. *Sociology of Health and Illness* 1990;**12**:336–50.

5 Introducing focus groups

JENNY KITZINGER

This chapter introduces focus group methodology, gives advice on group composition, running the groups, and analysing the results. Focus groups have advantages for researchers in the field of health and medicine: they do not discriminate against people who cannot read or write and they can encourage participation from people reluctant to be interviewed on their own or who feel they have nothing to say.

Rationale and uses of focus groups

Focus groups are a form of group interview that capitalises on communication between research participants in order to generate data. Although group interviews are often used simply as a quick and convenient way to collect data from several people simultaneously, the purpose of focus groups is explicitly to use group interaction as part of the method. This means that instead of the researcher asking each person to respond to a question in turn, people are encouraged to talk to one another: asking questions, exchanging anecdotes and commenting on each others' experiences and points of view.[1] The method is particularly useful for exploring people's knowledge and experiences and can be used to examine not only what people think but how they think and why they think that way.

Focus groups were originally used within communication studies to explore the effects of films and television programmes,[2] and are a popular method for assessing health education messages and examining public understandings of illness and of health behaviours.[3-7] They are widely used to examine people's experiences of disease and of health services[8 9] and are an effective technique for exploring the attitudes and needs of staff.[10 11]

The idea behind the focus group method is that group processes can help people to explore and clarify their views in ways that would be less easily accessible in a one to one interview. Group discussion is particularly appropriate when the interviewer has a series of open ended questions and wishes to encourage research participants to explore the issues of importance to them, in their own vocabulary, generating their own questions and pursuing their own priorities. When group dynamics work well the participants work alongside the researcher, taking the research in new and often unexpected directions.

Group work also helps researchers tap into the many different forms of communication that people use in day to day interaction, including jokes, anecdotes, teasing, and arguing. Gaining access to such variety of communication is useful because people's knowledge and attitudes are not entirely encapsulated in reasoned responses to direct questions. Everyday forms of communication may tell us as much, if not more, about what people know or experience. In this sense focus groups reach the parts that other methods cannot reach, revealing dimensions of understanding that often remain untapped by more conventional data collection techniques.

Tapping into such interpersonal communication is also important because this can highlight (sub)cultural values or group norms. Through analysing the operation of humour, consensus, and dissent and examining different types of narrative used within the group, the researcher can identify shared and common knowledge.[12] This makes focus groups a data collection technique particularly sensitive to cultural variables—which is why it is so often used in cross cultural research and work with ethnic minorities. It also makes them useful in studies examining why different sections of the population make differential use of health services.[13 14] For similar reasons focus groups are useful for studying dominant cultural values (for example, exposing dominant narratives about sexuality[15]) and for examining work place cultures—the ways in which, for example, staff cope with working with terminally ill patients or deal with the stresses of an accident and emergency department.

The downside of such group dynamics is that the articulation of group norms may silence individual voices of dissent. The presence of other research participants also compromises the confidentiality of the research session. For example, in group discussion with old people in long term residential care I found that some residents tried to prevent others from criticising staff—becoming agitated and repeatedly interrupting with cries of "you can't complain"; "the staff couldn't possibly be nicer." On the one hand, such interactions highlighted certain aspects of these people's experiences. In this case, it showed some residents' fear of being "punished" by staff for, in the words of one woman, "being cheeky." On the other hand, such group dynamics raise ethical issues (especially when the work is with "captive" populations) and may limit the usefulness of the data for certain purposes (Scottish Health Feedback, unpublished report).

However, it should not be assumed that groups are, by definition, inhibiting relative to the supposed privacy of an interview situation or that focus groups are inappropriate when researching sensitive topics. Quite the opposite may be true. Group work can actively facilitate the discussion of taboo topics because the less inhibited members of the group break the ice for shyer participants. Participants can also provide mutual support in expressing feelings that are common to their group but which they consider to deviate from mainstream culture (or the assumed culture of the researcher). This is particularly important when researching stigmatised or taboo experiences (for example, bereavement or sexual violence).

Focus group methods are also popular with those conducting action research and those concerned to "empower" research participants because the participants can become an active part of the process of analysis. Indeed, group participants may actually develop particular perspectives as a consequence of talking with other people who have similar experiences. For example, group dynamics can allow for a shift from personal, self blaming psychological explanations ("I'm stupid not to have understood what the doctor was telling me"; "I should have been stronger—I should have asked the right questions") to the exploration of structural solutions ("If we've all felt confused about what we've been told maybe having a leaflet would help, or what about being able to take away a tape recording of the consultation?").

Some researchers have also noted that group discussions can

generate more critical comments than interviews.[16] For example, Geis *et al,* in their study of the lovers of people with AIDS, found that there were more angry comments about the medical community in the group discussions than in the individual interviews: "perhaps the synergism of the group 'kept the anger going' and allowed each participant to reinforce another's vented feelings of frustration and rage."[17] A method that facilitates the expression of criticism and the exploration of different types of solutions is invaluable if the aim of research is to improve services. Such a method is especially appropriate when working with particular disempowered patient populations who are often reluctant to give negative feedback or may feel that any problems result from their own inadequacies.[19]

Conducting a focus group study

Sampling and group composition

Focus group studies can consist of anything between half a dozen to over fifty groups, depending on the aims of the project and the resources available. Most studies involve just a few groups, and some combine this method with other data collection techniques. Focus group discussion of a questionnaire is ideal for testing the phrasing of questions and is also useful in explaining or exploring survey results.[19 20]

Although it may be possible to work with a representative sample of a small population, most focus group studies use a theoretical sampling model (explained earlier in this book[21]) whereby participants are selected to reflect a range of the total study population or to test particular hypotheses. Imaginative sampling is crucial. Most people now recognise class or ethnicity as important variables, and it is also worth considering other variables. For example, when exploring women's experiences of maternity care or cervical smears it may be advisable to include groups of lesbians or women who were sexually abused as children.[22]

Most researchers recommend aiming for homogeneity within each group in order to capitalise on people's shared experiences. However, it can also be advantageous to bring together a diverse group (for example, from a range of professions) to maximise exploration of different perspectives within a group setting. However, it is important to be aware of how hierarchy within the group may affect the data (a nursing auxiliary, for example, is likely to be inhibited by the presence of a consultant from the same hospital).

The groups can be "naturally occurring" (for example, people who work together) or may be drawn together specifically for the research. Using pre-existing groups allows observation of fragments of interactions that approximate to naturally occurring data (such as might have been collected by participant observation). An additional advantage is that friends and colleagues can relate each other's comments to incidents in their shared daily lives. They may challenge each other on contradictions between what they profess to believe and how they actually behave (for example, "how about that time you didn't use a glove while taking blood from a patient?").

However, it would be naive to assume that group data are by definition "natural" in the sense that such interactions would have occurred without the group being convened for this purpose. Rather than assuming that sessions inevitably reflect everyday interactions (although sometimes they will), the group should be used to encourage people to engage with one another, formulate their ideas, and draw out the cognitive structures which previously have not been articulated.

Finally, it is important to consider the appropriateness of group work for different study populations and to think about how to overcome potential difficulties. Group work can facilitate collecting information from people who cannot read or write. The "safety in numbers factor" may also encourage the participation of those who are wary of an interviewer or who are anxious about talking.[23] However, group work can compound difficulties in communication if each person has a different disability. In the study assessing residential care for the elderly, I conducted a focus group that included one person who had impaired hearing, another with senile dementia, and a third with partial paralysis affecting her speech. This severely restricted interaction between research participants and confirmed some of the staff's predictions about the limitations of group work with this population. However, such problems could be resolved by thinking more carefully about the composition of the group, and sometimes group participants could help to translate for each other. It should also be noted that some of the old people who might have been unable to sustain a one to one interview were able to take part in the group, contributing intermittently. Even some residents who staff had suggested should

> ## Some potential sampling advantages with focus groups
>
> - Do not discriminate against people who cannot read or write
> - Can encourage participation from those who are reluctant to be interviewed on their own (such as those intimidated by the formality and isolation of a one to one interview)
> - Can encourage contributions from people who feel they have nothing to say or who are deemed "unresponsive patients" (but engage in the discussion generated by other group members)

be excluded from the research because they were "unresponsive" eventually responded to the lively conversations generated by other residents and were able to contribute their point of view. Communication difficulties should not rule out group work, but must be considered as a factor.

Running the groups

Sessions should be relaxed: a comfortable setting, refreshments, and sitting round in a circle will help to establish the right atmosphere. The ideal group size is between four and eight people. Sessions may last one to two hours (or extend into a whole afternoon or a series of meetings). The facilitator should explain that the aim of focus groups is to encourage people to talk to each other rather than to address themselves to the researcher. The researcher may take a back seat at first, allowing for a type of "structured eavesdropping."[24] Later on in the session, however, the researcher can adopt a more interventionist style: urging debate to continue beyond the stage it might otherwise have ended and guiding the group to discuss the inconsistencies both between participants and within their own thinking. Disagreements within groups can be used to encourage participants to elucidate their point of view and to clarify why they think as they do. Differences between individual one off interviews have to be analysed by the researchers through armchair theorising; differences between members of focus groups should be explored in situ with the help of the research participants.

The facilitator may also use a range of group exercises. A common exercise consists of presenting the group with a series of statements on large cards. The group members are asked collectively to sort these cards into different piles depending on, for example, their degree of agreement or disagreement with that point of view or the importance they assign to that particular aspect of service. For example, I have used such cards to explore public understandings of HIV transmission (placing statements about "types" of people into different risk categories), old people's experiences of residential care (assigning degrees of importance to different statements about the quality of their care), and midwives' views of their professional responsibilities (placing a series of statements about midwives' roles along an agree-disagree continuum). Such exercises encourage participants to concentrate on one another (rather than on the group facilitator) and force them to explain their different perspectives. The final layout of the cards is less important than the discussion that it generates.[25] Researchers may also use such exercises as a way of checking out their own assessment of what has emerged from the group. In this case it is best to take along a series of blank cards and fill them out only towards the end of the session, using statements generated during the course of the discussion. Finally, it may be beneficial to present research participants with a brief questionnaire, or the opportunity to speak to the researcher individually, giving each one the chance to record private comments after the group session has been completed.

Ideally the group discussions should be tape recorded and transcribed. If this is not possible then it is vital to take careful notes and researchers may find it useful to involve the group in recording key issues on a flip chart.

Analysis and writing up

Analysing focus groups is basically the same as analysing any other qualitative self report data.[21 26] At the very least, the researcher draws together and compares discussions of similar themes and examines how these relate to the variables within the sample population. In general, it is not appropriate to give percentages in reports of focus group data, and it is important to try to distinguish between individual opinions expressed in spite of the group from the actual group consensus. As in all qualitative analysis, deviant case analysis is important—that is, attention must be given to minority opinions and examples that do not fit with the researcher's overall theory.

The only distinct feature of working with focus group data is the need to indicate the impact of the group dynamic and analyse the sessions in ways that take full advantage of the interaction between research participants. In coding the script of a group discussion, it is worth using special categories for certain types of narrative, such as jokes and anecdotes, and types of interaction, such as "questions," "deferring to the opinion of others," "censorship," or "changes of mind." A focus group research report that is true to its data should also usually include at least some illustration of the talk between participants, rather than simply presenting isolated quotations taken out of context.

Conclusion

This chapter has presented the factors to consider when designing or evaluating a focus group study. In particular, it has drawn attention to the overt exploitation and exploration of interactions in focus group discussion. Interaction between participants can be used to achieve seven main aims:

• To highlight the respondents' attitudes, priorities, language, and framework of understanding
• To encourage research participants to generate and explore their own questions and develop their own analysis of common experiences
• To encourage a variety of communication from participants—tapping into a wide range and form of understanding
• To help to identify group norms and cultural values
• To provide insight into the operation of group social processes in the articulation of knowledge (for example, through the examination of what information is censured or muted within the group)
• To encourage open conversation about embarrassing subjects and to permit the expression of criticism
• Generally to facilitate the expression of ideas and experiences that might be left underdeveloped in an interview and to illuminate the research participants' perspectives through the debate within the group.

Group data are neither more nor less authentic than data collected by other methods, but focus groups can be the most appropriate method for researching particular types of question. Direct observation may be more appropriate for studies of social roles and formal organisation[27] but focus groups are particularly suited to the study of attitudes and experiences. Interviews may be more appropriate for tapping into individual biographies,[27] but focus groups are more suitable for examining how knowledge, and more importantly, ideas, develop and operate within a given cultural context. Questionnaires are more appropriate for obtaining quantitative information and explaining how many people hold a certain (pre-defined) opinion; focus groups are better for exploring exactly how those opinions are constructed. Thus while surveys repeatedly identify gaps between health knowledge and health behaviour, only qualitative methods, such as focus groups, can actually fill these gaps and explain why these occur.

Focus groups are not an easy option. The data they generate can be as cumbersome as they are complex. Yet the method is basically straightforward and need not be intimidating for either the researcher or the researched. Perhaps the very best way of working out whether or not focus groups might be appropriate in any particular study is to try them out in practice.

Further reading

Morgan D. *Focus groups as qualitative research*. London: Sage, 1988.
Kreuger R. *Focus groups: a practical guide for applied research*. London: Sage, 1988.

1 Kitzinger J. The methodology of focus groups: the importance of interactions between research participants. *Sociology of Health and Illness* 1994;16:103–21.
2 Merton R, Fisk M, Kendall P. *The focused interview: a report of the bureau of applied social research*. New York: Columbia University, 1956.
3 Basch C. Focus group interview: an under-utilised research technique for improving theory and practice in health education. *Health Education Quarterly* 1987;14:411–8.
4 Kitzinger J. Understanding AIDS: researching audience perceptions of acquired immune deficiency syndrome. In Eldridge J, ed. *Getting the message: news, truth and power*. London: Routledge, 1993:271–305.
5 Ritchie JE, Herscovitch F, Norfor JB. Beliefs of blue collar workers regarding coronary risk behaviours. *Health Education Research* 1994;9:95–103.
6 Duke SS, Gordon-Sosby, K, Reynolds, KD, Gram IT. A study of breast cancer detection practices and beliefs in black women attending public health clinics. *Health Education Research* 1994;9:331–42.
7 Khan M, Manderson L. Focus groups in tropical diseases research. *Health Policy and Planning* 1992;7:56–66.
8 Murray S, Tapson J, Turnbull L, McCallum J, Little A. Listening to local voices: adapting rapid appraisal to assess health and social needs in general practice. *BMJ* 1994;308:698–700.
9 Gregory S, McKie L. The smear test: listening to women's views. *Nursing Standard* 1991;5:32–6.
10 Brown J, Lent B, Sas G. Identifying and treating wife abuse. *Journal of Family Practice* 1993;36:185–91.
11 Denning JD, Verschelden C. Using the focus group in assessing training needs: empowering child welfare workers. *Child Welfare* 1993;72:569–79.
12 Hughes D, Dumont K. Using focus groups to facilitate culturally anchored research. *American Journal of Community Psychology* 1993; 21:775–806.
13 Zimmerman M, Haffey J, Crane E, Szumowski D, Alvarez F, Bhiromrut P, *et al.* Assessing

the acceptability of NORPLANT implants in four countries: findings from focus group research. *Studies in Family Planning* 1990;21:92–103.

14 Naish J, Brown J, Denton B. Intercultural consultations: investigation of factors that deter non-English speaking women from attending their general practitioners for cervical screening. *BMJ* 1994;309:1126–8.

15 Barker G, Rich S. Influences on adolescent sexuality in Nigeria and Kenya: findings from recent focus-group discussions. *Studies in Family Planning* 1992;23:199–210.

16 Watts M, Ebbutt D. More than the sum of the parts: research methods in group interviewing. *British Educational Research Journal* 1987;13:25–34.

17 Geis S, Fuller R, Rush J. Lovers of AIDS victims: psychosocial stresses and counselling needs. *Death Studies* 1986;10:43–53.

18 DiMatteo M, Khan K, Berry S. Narratives of birth and the postpartum: an analysis of the focus group responses of new mothers. *Birth* 1993;20:204.

19 Kitzinger J. Focus groups: method or madness? In Boulton M, ed. *Challenge and innovation: methodological advances in social research on HIV/AIDS.* London: Taylor and Francis, 1994:159–75.

20 O'Brien K. Improving survey questionnaires through focus groups. In Morgan D, ed. *Successful focus groups: advancing the state of the art.* London: Sage, 1993:105–18.

21 Mays N, Pope C. Rigour and qualitative research. *BMJ* 1995;311:109–12.

22 Kitzinger J. Recalling the pain: incest survivors' experiences of obstetrics and gynaecology. *Nursing Times* 1990;86:38–40.

23 Lederman L. High apprehensives talk about communication apprehension and its effects on their behaviour. *Communication Quarterly* 1983;31:233–37.

24 Powney J. Structured eavesdropping. *Research Intelligence (Journal of the British Educational Research Foundation)* 1988;28:10–2.

25 Kitzinger J. Audience understanding AIDS: a discussion of methods. *Sociology of Health and Illness* 1990;12:319–35.

26 Britten N. Qualitative interviews in medical research. *BMJ* 1995;311:251–3.

27 Mays N, Pope C. Observational methods in health care settings. *BMJ* 1995;311:182–4.

6 Consensus methods for medical and health services research

JEREMY JONES, DUNCAN HUNTER

Health providers face the problem of trying to make decisions in situations where there is insufficient information and also where there is an overload of (often contradictory) information. Statistical methods such as meta-analysis have been developed to summarise and to resolve inconsistencies in study finding—where information is available in an appropriate form. Consensus methods provide another means of synthesising information, but are liable to use a wider range of information than is common in statistical methods, and where published information is inadequate or non-existent these methods provide a means of harnessing the insights of appropriate experts to enable decisions to be made. Two consensus methods commonly adopted in medical, nursing, and health services research— the Delphi process and the nominal group technique (also known as the expert panel)—are described, together with the most appropriate situations for using them; an outline of the process involved in undertaking a study using each method is supplemented by illustrations of the authors' work. Key methodological issues in using the methods are discussed, along with the distinct contribution of consensus methods as aids to decision making, both in clinical practice and in health service development.

Box 1—Features of consensus methods

Anonymity	To avoid dominance; achieved by use of a questionnaire in Delphi and private ranking in nominal group
Iteration	Processes occur in "rounds", allowing individuals to change their opinions
Controlled feedback	Showing the distribution of the group's response (indicating to each individual their own previous response in Delphi)
Statistical group response	Expressing judgment using summary measures of the full group response, giving more information than just a consensus statement

Adapted from Pill[1] and Rowe[2]

Defining consensus and consensus methods

Quantitative methods such as meta-analysis have been developed to provide statistical overviews of the results of clinical trials and to resolve inconsistencies in the results of published studies. Consensus methods are another means of dealing with conflicting scientific evidence. They allow a wider range of study types to be considered than is usual in statistical reviews. In addition they allow a greater role for the quantitative assessment of evidence (box 1). These methods, unlike those described in the other papers in this series, are primarily concerned with deriving quantitative estimates through qualitative approaches.

The aim of consensus methods is to determine the extent to which experts or lay people agree about a given issue. They seek to overcome some of the disadvantages normally found with decision making in groups or committees, which are commonly dominated by one individual or by coalitions representing vested interests. In open committees individuals are often not ready to retract long held and publicly stated opinions, even when these have been proved to be false.

The term "agreement" takes two forms, which need to be distinguished: firstly, the extent to which each respondent agrees with the issue under consideration (typically rated on a numerical or categorical scale) and, secondly, the extent to which respondents

47

agree with each other, the consensus element of these studies (typically assessed by statistical measures of average and dispersion).

Application

The focus of consensus methods lies where unanimity of opinion does not exist owing to a lack of scientific evidence or where there is contradictory evidence on an issue. The methods attempt to assess the extent of agreement (consensus measurement) and to resolve disagreement (consensus development).

The three best known consensus methods are the Delphi process, the nominal group technique (also known as the expert panel), and the consensus development conference. Each of these methods involves measuring consensus, and the last two methods are also concerned with developing consensus. The consensus development conference will not be covered in this chapter because it requires resources beyond those at the disposal of most researchers (unlike the other two methods), is commonly organised within defined programmes (for example, by the King's Fund in Britain and the National Institutes of Health in the United States), and has been discussed at length elsewhere.[3-6]

The methods described

The Delphi process

The Delphi process takes its name from the Delphic oracle's skills of interpretation and foresight and proceeds in a series of rounds as follows:

● Round 1: Either the relevant individuals are invited to provide opinions on a specific matter, based on their knowledge and experience, or the team undertaking the Delphi expresses opinions on a specific matter and selects suitable experts to participate in subsequent questionnaire rounds
● These opinions are grouped together under a limited number of headings and statements drafted for circulation to all participants on a questionnaire
● Round 2: Participants rank their agreement with each statement in the questionnaire
● The rankings are summarised and included in a repeat version of the questionnaire
● Round 3: Participants rerank their agreement with each state-

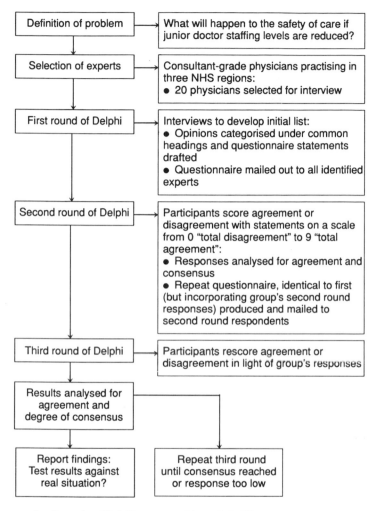

FIGURE 1—*Examples of Delphi process used in study by JJ.*

ment in the questionnaire, with the opportunity to change their score in view of the group's response

• The rerankings are summarised and assessed for degree of consensus: if an acceptable degree of consensus is obtained the process may cease, with final results fed back to participants; if not, the third round is repeated.

Figure 1 shows an example of this process for a Delphi study undertaken by one of the authors (JJ). In addition to scoring agreement with statements, respondents are commonly asked to rate the confidence or certainty with which they express their opinions.

The Delphi technique has been used widely in health research within the fields of technology assessment,[7-10] education and training[11-14] and priorities and information,[15-17] and in developing nursing and clinical practice.[19-21] It enables a large group of experts to be contacted cheaply, usually by mail with a self administered questionnaire (though computer communications have also been used), with few geographical limitations on the sample. Some situations have included a round in which the participants meet to discuss the process and resolve uncertainty or any ambiguities in the wording of the questionnaire.

The nominal group technique

The nominal group technique uses a highly structured meeting to gather information from relevant experts (usually 9–12 in number) about a given issue. It consists of two rounds in which panellists rate, discuss, and then rerate a series of items or questions. The method was developed in the United States in the 1960s and has been applied to problems in social services, education, government, and industry.[22] In the context of health care the method has most commonly been used to examine the appropriateness of clinical interventions[23-27] but has also been applied in education and training,[28-30] in practice development,[31-33] and for identifying measures for clinical trials.[34-36]

A nominal group meeting is facilitated either by an expert on the topic[37] or a credible non-expert[38] and is structured as follows:

- Participants spend several minutes writing down their views about the topic in question
- Each participant, in turn, contributes one idea to the facilitator, who records it on a flip chart
- Similar suggestions are grouped together, where appropriate. There is a group discussion to clarify and evaluate each idea
- Each participant privately ranks each idea (round 1)
- The ranking is tabulated and presented
- The overall ranking is discussed and reranked (round 2)
- The final rankings are tabulated and the results fed back to participants.

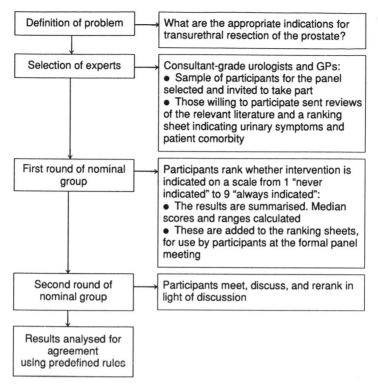

FIGURE 2—*Example of modified nominal group undertaken by DH*

Figure 2 shows an example of a modified nominal group undertaken by one of the authors (DH).

The method can be adapted and has been conducted as a single meeting or with the first stage conducted by post followed by a discussion and rerating at a face to face meeting. Some nominal group meetings have incorporated a detailed review of literature as background material for the topic under discussion.

Alongside the consensus process there may be a non-participant observer collecting qualitative data on the nominal group. This approach has some features in common with focus groups (see Chapter 5). However, the nominal group technique focuses on a single goal (for example, the definition of criteria to assess the appropriateness of a surgical intervention) and is less concerned with eliciting a range of ideas or the qualitative analysis of the group process per se than is the case in focus groups.

Methodological issues

Who to include as participants

There can be few hard and fast rules about who to include as participants, except that each must be justifiable as in some way "expert" on the matter under discussion. Clearly, for studies concerned with defining criteria for clinical intervention, the most appropriate experts will be clinicians practising in the field under consideration. However, the inclusion of other clinicians such as general practitioners may be appropriate to provide an alternative clinical view, particularly when the study is expected to have an impact beyond a particular specialist field. When the discussion concerns matters of general interest, such as health service priorities, participants should include non-clinical health professionals and the expression of lay opinions should also be allowed for.

There is clearly a potential for bias in the selection of participants. Although it has been shown that doctors who are willing to participate in expert panels are representative of their colleagues,[40] the exact composition of the panel can affect the results obtained.[24] The results will also be affected by any "random" variation in panel behaviour. These problems can be overcome by using a different mixture of participants in further panels.

How to measure the accuracy of the answer obtained

The existence of a consensus does not mean that the "correct" answer has been found—there is the danger of deriving collective ignorance rather than wisdom. The nominal group is not a replacement for rigorous scientific reviews of published reports or for original research, but rather a means of identifying current medical opinion and areas of disagreement. For Delphi surveys, Pill recommends that the results should, when possible, be matched to observable events.[1] Observers of the accuracy of opinion polls before the 1992 general election in Britain might well agree with this conclusion.

How to feed back the results of each round

Agreement with statements is usually summarised by using the median and consensus assessed by using interquartile ranges for continuous numerical scales. These summary statistics may be fed

Box 2—Example of feedback of second round results in a Delphi[40]

The following are possible adverse effects of lowering the number of junior medical staff in general medicine and its associated specialties. The star indicates the number you selected to indicate the extent to which you agreed or disagreed with each statement in response to the previous questionnaire. Each of the numbers below the scale represents the percentage of those responding to the questionnaire who selected that particular value. We would be grateful if you would read through the questionnaire and consider whether, in the light of your colleagues' assessments, you would like to alter your response. Please indicate the extent to which you agree or disagree with each statement by circling the appropriate number (0 indicates total disagreement and 9 total agreement): if your choice remains unchanged please circle the same number you selected on the previous questionnaire.

i) Mortality rates in hospital will rise

```
                             *
         _____
disagree  0 1 2 3 4  5  6  7  8  9  agree
          5–3–9–4–3–18–18–12–16–12
```

back to participants at each round along with fuller indications of the distribution of responses to each statement in the form of tables of the proportions ranking at each point on the scale (see box 2), histograms, or other graphical representations of the range (see box 3). Feeding back the group's response enables participants to consider their initial ranking in relation to their colleagues' assessments. It should be made clear to each participant that they need not conform to the group view—though, in the nominal group technique, those with atypical opinions (compared with the rest of the group) may face critical questioning of their view from other panel members. In a Delphi exercise, the researcher undertaking the study may ask participants who they have defined as outliers (for example, those in the lower and upper quartiles) to provide written justification for their responses.

For nominal groups, rules have been developed to assess agreement when statements have been ranked on a 9 point scale (see box 3). In this example, the scale can be broken down so that scores 1–3 represent a region where participants feel intervention is not indicated; 4–6, a region where participants are equivocal; and

---

Box 3—Example of feedback of first round results in a nominal group[23]

A—Chronic Retention: TURP is indicated for patients with chronic retention (but not acute) and there are:

IRRITATIVE SYMPTOMS

	High	Medium	Low
None	1②3 4 5 6 7 8 9	1 2③4 5 6 7 8 9	1 2 3④5 6 7 8 9
Mild	1②3 4 5 6 7 8 9	1 2⑤4 5 6 7 8 9	1 2 3 4⑤6 7 8 9
Moderate	1 2 3④5 6 7 8 9	1 2 3 4 5⑥7 8 9	1 2 3 4 5 6⑦8 9
Severe	1 2 3 4 5⑥7 8 9	1 2 3 4 5 6 7⑧9	1 2 3 4 5 6 7 8⑨

1 never indicated; 2 always indicated; ○ median; — range.

Box 4—Examples of strict and relaxed rules for agreement in a nominal group

1②3 4 5 6 7 8 9	Strict:	all ratings fall within a predefined 3 point region (agreement that intervention is "not indicated")
1 ②3 4 5 6 7 8 9	Relaxed:	all ratings fall within a 3 point region, but not one of the predefined regions (crossing "not indicated" (1–3) and "equivocal" (4-6) regions

---

7–9, a region where participants feel intervention is indicated. The first rule is based on where the scores fall on the ranking scale (box 4): if all ratings fall within one of these predefined regions there is said to be strict agreement (in the example, all participants agreed that transurethral resection of the prostate was not indicated). An alternative relaxed definition for agreement is that all ratings fall within any 3 point region. This may be treated as agreement, in that all ratings are within an acceptable range, but the group opinion is ambiguous as to whether intervention is indicated or not.

The second rule tests whether extreme rankings are having an undue influence on the final results and consists of assessing the strict and relaxed definitions by including all ratings for each statement and then by excluding one extreme high and one extreme low rating for each statement. The ranges indicated in box

3 include all ratings, and it is noticeable that several of these ranges are from 1 to 9. It may be that these ranges exaggerate the dispersion of the group's response.

Validity and applicability

There has been an active debate on the validity of the Delphi method. For example, Harold Sackman argued that the Delphi method fails to meet the standards normally set for scientific methods.[41] Many of his criticisms were aimed at past studies of poor quality rather than fundamental critiques of the method itself; he particularly criticised poor questionnaire design, inadequate testing of reliability and validity of methods, and the methods of defining and selecting experts. He also argued that the method forces consensus and is weakened by not allowing participants to discuss issues.

Reviews by Pill[1] and by Gerth and Smith (personal communication) showed no clear evidence in favour of meeting based methods over Delphi. Rowe *et al*, though, concluded that the Delphi technique is generally inferior to the nominal group technique, but state that the degree of inferiority is small, arising more from practical than from theoretical difficulties; they argue for further research aiming to improve the practice of Delphi studies—particularly a careful consideration of what constitutes expertise.[2]

Consensus methods, in particular Delphi, have been described as methods of "last resort,"[42] with defenders warning against "overselling" the methods[43] and suggesting that they should be regarded more as methods for structuring group communication than as a means for providing answers. There is clearly a danger that since these approaches have a prescribed method and are often used to generate quantitative estimates, they may lead the casual observer to place greater reliance on their results than might be warranted. As we stated earlier, unless the findings can be tested against observed data, we can never be sure that the methods have produced the "correct" answer. This should be made clear in reporting study results.

The structures of Delphi and nominal groups (shown in box 1) aim to maximise the benefits from having informed panels consider a problem (often termed "process gain") while minimising the disadvantages associated with collective decision making ("process loss"), particularly domination by individuals or professional interests. The extent to which these realised depends on the ability of those running the studies to use the advantages of the methods. An important role of the facilitator in the nominal group is to ensure that all participants are able to express their views and to keep particular personal or professional views from dominating the discussion; participants in both Delphi and nominal group panels should be selected as to ensure that no particular interest or preconceived opinion is likely to dominate.

Uses

Consensus methods provide a useful way of identifying and measuring uncertainty in medical and health services research. Delphi and nominal group techniques have been used to clarify particular issues in health service organisation: to define professional roles, to aid design of educational programmes, to enable long term projections of need for care for particular client groups where there has been considerable uncertainty (for example, for cases of HIV and AIDS[9]), and to develop criteria for appropriateness of interventions as part of technology assessment. In addition to forming studies in their own right, these techniques have been widely used as component parts of larger projects.[8 31] The two pieces of research from which materials have been presented in this paper each formed part of larger projects: the Delphi exercise[44] was concerned with defining possible adverse effects of reducing junior doctors staffing levels as part of a study of the adequacy of hospital medical staffing levels; the nominal group[23] was concerned with defining appropriate indications for surgical intervention as part of a population based assessment of need for prostate surgery within an NHS region.

Conclusions

The emphasis, when the findings of Delphi and nominal group studies are presented, should be on the justification in using such methods, the use of sound methodology (including selection of experts and the clear definition of target "acceptable" levels of consensus), appropriate presentation of findings (where proposed standards for presentation—as for clinical practice guidelines[45]— should be considered), and on the relevance and systematic use of the results. The output from consensus approaches (including consensus development conferences) is rarely an end in itself.

Dissemination and implementation of such findings is the ultimate aim of consensus activities—for example, the publication of consensus statements intended to guide health policy, clinical practice, and research, such as the consensus statement on cancer of the colon and rectum.[46]

Further reading

Fink A, Kosecoff J, Chassin M, Brook R. Consensus methods: characteristics and guidelines for use. *Am J Public Health* 1984;74:979–83.

1 Pill J. The Delphi method: substance, context, a critique and an annotated bibliography. *Socio-Economic Planning Science* 1971;5:57–71.
2 Rowe G, Wright B, Bolger F. Delphi: a re-evaluation of research and theory. *Technological Forecasting and Social Change* 1991;39:235–51.
3 McGlynn EA, Kosecoff J, Brook RH. Format and conduct of consensus development conferences. *International Journal of Technology Assessment in Health Care* 1990;6:450–69.
4 Perry S. The NIH consensus development program: a decade later. *N Engl J Med* 1987;317:485–8.
5 Perry S, Kalberer JT. The NIH consensus development program and the assessment of health care technologies: the first two years. *N Engl J Med* 1980;303:169–72.
6 Stocking B, Jennet B, Spiby J. Criteria for change. In: *The history and impact of consensus development conferences in the UK.* London: King's Fund Centre, 1991.
7 Beers MH, Ouslander JG, Rollinger I, Reuben DB, Brooks J, Beck JC. Explicit criteria for determining inappropriate use in nursing home residents. *Arch Intern Med* 1991;151:1825–32.
8 Bellamy N, Anastassiades TP, Buchanan WW, Davis L, Lee P, McCain GA, *et al.* Rheumatoid arthritis anti-rheumatic trials. III. Setting the delta for clinical trials of anti-rheumatic drugs—results of a consensus development (Delphi) exercise. *J Rheumatol* 1991;18:1908–15.
9 Chin J, Sato PA, Mann JM. Projections of HIV infections and AIDS cases to the year 2000. *Bull World Health Organ* 1990;68:1–11.
10 Khan JP, Bernstein SJ, Leape LL, Hilborne LH, Park RE, Parker L, *et al.* Measuring the necessity of medical procedures. *Med Care* 1994;32:357–65.
11 Crotty M. The emerging role of the British nurse teacher in Project 2000 programmes: a Delphi survey. *J Adv Nurs* 1993;18:150–7.
12 Fraser CE, Smith QW, Luchi RJ. Geriatric fellows' perceptions of the quality of their research training. *Acad Med* 1992;67:696–8.
13 Elder OC Jr, Andrew ME. Important curriculum content for baccalaureate allied health programs: a survey of deans. *J Allied Health* 1992;21:105–15.
14 Rizzolo MA. Factors influencing the development and use of interactive video in nursing education. A Delphi study. *Comput Nurs* 1990;8:151–9.
15 Attala JM, Gresley RS, McSweeney N, Jobe MA. Health needs of school-age children in two midwestern counties. *Issues in Comprehensive Paediatric Nursing* 1993;16:51–60.
16 Moscovice I, Armstrong P, Shortell S. Health services research for decision-makers: the use of the Delphi technique to determine health priorities. *J. Health Polit Policy Law* 1988;2:388–410.
17 Oranga HM, Nordeberg E. The Delphi panel method for generating health information. *Health Policy and Planning* 1993;8:405–12.
18 Rainhorn JD, Brudon-Jakobowicz P, Reich MR. Priorities for pharmaceutical policies in developing countries: results of a Delphi survey. *Bull World Health Organ* 1994;72:257–64.
19 Mobily PR, Herr KA, Kelley LS. Cognitive-behavioural techniques to reduce pain: a validation study. *Int J Nurs Stud* 1993;30:537–48.
20 Passannante MR, Restifo RA, Reichman LB. Preventive therapy for the patient with both universal indication and contraindication for isoniazid. *Chest* 1993;103:825–31.

21 Smith DM, Murphy WM. Histological changes in prostate carcinomas treated with leuprolide (luteinizing hormone-releasing hormone effect). Distinction from tumor differentiation. *Cancer* 1994;73:1472–7.
22 Fink A, Kosecoff J, Chassin M, Brook RH. Consensus methods: characteristics and guidelines for use. *Am J Public Health* 1984;74:979–83.
23 Hunter DJW, McKee CM, Sanderson CFB, Black NA. Appropriateness of prostatectomy: a consensus panel approach. *J Epidemiol Community Health* 1994;48:58–64.
24 Scott EA, Black NA. Appropriateness of cholecystectomy—a consensus panel approach. *Gut* 1991;9:1066–70.
25 Technology Subcommittee of the Working Group on Critical Care, Ontario Ministry of Health. Hemodynamic monitoring: a technology assessment. *Can Med Assoc J* 1991;145:114–21.
26 Technology Subcommittee of the Working Group on Critical Care, Ontario Ministry of Health: Guidelines for medical technology in critical care. *Can Med Assoc J* 1991;144:1617–22.
27 Ziemba SE, Hubbell FA, Fine MJ, Burns MJ. Resting electrocardiograms as baseline tests: impact on the management of elderly patients. *Am J Med* 1991;91:576–83.
28 Battles JB, Kirk LM, Dowell DL, Frnka S. The health sciences communicator as faculty developer. *J Biocommun* 1989;16:2–8.
29 Buchan MS, Hegge MJ, Stenvig TE. A tiger by the tail: tackling barriers to differentiated practice. *J Contin Educ Nurse* 1991;22:109–12.
30 McKee M, Priest P, Ginzler M, Black N. What tasks performed by pre-registration house officers out of hours are appropriate? *Med Educ* 1992;23:51–7.
31 Justice J, Jang R. Tapping employee insights with the Nominal Group Technique. *Am Pharm* 1990;NS30:43–5.
32 Manning D, Balson PM, Barenberg N, Moore TM. Susceptibility to AIDS; what college students do and don't believe. *J Am Coll Health* 1989;38:67–73.
33 Neidlinger SH, Ljutic PM, Moed AB, Chin PP, Kowalczyk ME, Anton RS. Defining the major nursing administration issue: doing more with less. *J Nurs Admin* 1993;23:9–10.
34 Felson DT. Choosing a core set of disease activity measures for rheumatoid arthritis clinical trials. *J Rheumatol* 1993;20:531–4.
35 Gallagher M, Hares T, Spencer J, Bradshaw C, Webb I. The nominal group technique: a research tool for general practice? *Fam Pract* 1993;10:76–81.
36 Liang MH, Katz JN, Phillips C, Sledge C, Cats-Baril W. The total hip arthroplasty outcome evaluation form of the American Academy of Orthopaedic Surgeons. Results of a nominal group process. The American Academy of Orthopaedic Surgeons Task Force on Outcome Studies. *J Bone Joint Surg [AM]* 1991;73:639–46.
37 Delbeq A, Van de Ven A. A group process model for problem identification and program planning. *Journal of Applied Behavioural Science* 1971;7:467–92.
38 Glaser EM. Using behavioural science strategies for defining the state-of-the-art. *Journal of Applied and Behavioural Sciences* 1980;16:79–92.
39 Kitzinger J. Introducing focus groups. *BMJ* 1995;311:299–302.
40 McKee M, Priest P, Ginzler M, Black N. How representative are members of expert panels? *Quality Assurance in Health Care* 1991;3:89–94.
41 Sackman H. *Delphi critique*. Lexington, MA: Lexington Books, 1975.
42 Coates JF. In defense of Delphi: a review of *Delphi assessment, expert opinion, forecasting and group process* by H Sackman. *Technological Forecasting and Social Change* 1975;7:193–4.
43 Linstone HA. The Delphi technique. In: Fowles RB, ed. *Handbook of futures research*. Westport, CT: Greenwood, 1978.
44 Jones JMG, Sanderson CFB, Black NA. What will happen to the quality of care with fewer junior doctors? A Delphi study of consultant physicians' views. *J R Coll Physicians Lond* 1992;26:36–40.
45 Hayward RSA, Wilson MC, Tunis SR, Bass EB, Rubin HR, Haynes RB. More informative abstract of articles describing clinical practice guidelines. *Ann Intern Med* 1993;118:731–7.
46 King's Fund Forum. Consensus statement on cancer of the colon and rectum. *Int J Technol Assess Health Care* 1991;7:236–9.

7 Case study evaluation

JUSTIN KEEN, TIM PACKWOOD

Case study evaluations, using one or more qualitative methods, have been used to investigate important practical and policy questions in health care. This chapter describes the features of a well designed case study and gives examples showing how qualitative methods are used in evaluations of health services and health policy.

Introduction

The medical approach to understanding disease has traditionally drawn heavily on qualitative data, and in particular on case studies to illustrate important or interesting phenomena. The tradition continues today, not least in regular case reports in medical journals. Moreover, much of the everyday work of doctors and other health professionals still involves decisions that are qualitative rather than quantitative in nature.

This chapter discusses the use of qualitative research methods, not in clinical care but in case study evaluations of health service interventions. It is useful for doctors to understand the principles guiding the design and conduct of these evaluations, because they are frequently used by both researchers and inspectorial agencies (such as the Audit Commission in the United Kingdom and the General Accounting Office in the United States) to investigate the work of doctors and other health professionals.

We briefly discuss the circumstances in which case study research can usefully be undertaken in health service settings and the ways in which qualitative methods are used within case studies. Examples show how qualitative methods are applied, both in purely qualitative studies and alongside quantitative methods.

Case study evaluations

Doctors often find themselves asking important practical questions, such as should we be involved in the management of hospitals and, if so, how? How will new government policies effect the lives of our patients? And, how can we cope with changes in practice in our local setting? There are, broadly, two ways in which such questions can usefully be addressed. One is to analyse the proposed policies themselves, by investigating whether they are internally consistent and by using theoretical frameworks to predict their effects on the ground. National policies, including the implementation of the NHS internal market[1] and the new community care arrangements[2] have been examined in this way by using economic and other theories to analyse their likely consequences.

The other approach, and the focus of this chapter, is to study implementation empirically. Empirical evaluative studies are concerned with placing a value on an intervention or policy change, and they typically involve forming judgments, firstly about the appropriateness of an intervention for those concerned (and often by implication also for the NHS as a whole) and, secondly about whether the outputs and outcomes of interventions are justified by their inputs and processes.

Case study evaluations are valuable where broad, complex questions have to be addressed in complex circumstances. No one method is sufficient to capture all salient aspects of an intervention, and case studies typically use multiple methods.

The methods used in case studies may be qualitative or quantitative, depending on the circumstances. Case studies using qualitative methods are most valuable when the question being posed requires an investigation of a real life intervention in detail, where the focus is on how and why the intervention succeeds or fails, where the general context will influence the outcome and where researchers asking the questions will have no control over events. As a result, the number of relevant variables will be far greater than can be controlled for, so that experimental approaches are simply not appropriate.

Other conditions that enhance the value of the case study approach concern the nature of the intervention being investigated. Often an intervention is ill defined, at least at the outset, and so cannot easily be distinguished from the general environment. Even where it is well defined, an intervention may not be discrete but consist of a complete mix of changes that occur over different timescales. This is a pervasive problem in health services in many countries, which are experiencing many parallel and interrelated changes. The doctor weighing up whether or how to become involved in hospital management would have to assess the various impacts on the managerial role of clinical audit, resource management, consultant job plans, and a raft of government legislation. Secondly, any intervention will typically depend for its success on the involvement of several different interested groups. Each group may have a legitimate, but different, interpretation of events; capturing these different views is often best achieved by using interviews or other qualitative methods within a case study design. Thirdly, it is not clear at the outset whether an intervention will be fully implemented by the end of a study period—accounts of major computer system failures show this.[3] Yet study of these failures may provide invaluable clues for future success.

Taken together, these conditions exclude experimental approaches to evaluation. The case study is an alternative approach—in effect, a different way of thinking about complex situations which takes the conditions into account, but is nevertheless rigorous and facilitates informed judgments about success or failure.

The design of case studies

As noted earlier, case studies using qualitative methods are used by bodies that inspect and regulate public services. Examples include the work of the National Audit Office and the Audit Commission[4] in the United Kingdom and the Office of Technology Assessment in the United States.[5] Sometimes these studies are retrospective, particularly in investigations of failed implementations of policies. Increasingly, though, these bodies use prospective studies designed to investigate the extent to which centrally determined standards or initiatives have been implemented. For example, the National Audit Office recently examined hospital catering in England, focusing on the existence of, and monitoring of, standards as required by the citizen's charter and on the application of central policy and guidance in the areas of nutritional standards and cost control.[6]

Prospective studies have also been used by academic researchers, for example, to evaluate the introduction of general management[7] in Britain after the Griffiths report,[8] in the studies of specific changes following the 1989 NHS review[9] which were commissioned by the King's Fund,[10] and in the introduction of total quality management in hospitals in the United States.[11] In these cases the investigators were interested in understanding what happened in a complex environment where they had no control over events. Their research questions emerged from widespread concerns about the implications of new policies or management theories, and were investigated with the most appropriate methods at their disposal.

The nature of research questions

Once a broad research question has been identified, there are two approaches to the design of case study research, with appropriateness depending on the circumstances. In the first approach, precise questions are posed at the outset of the research and data collection and analysis are directed towards answering them. These studies are typically constructed to allow comparisons to be drawn.[12] The comparison may be between different approaches to implementation, or a comparison between sites where an intervention is taking place and ones where normal practice prevails.

An example is the recent study by Glennerster et al of the implementation of general practitioner fundholding.[13] Starting with a broad question about the value of general practitioner fundholding, the researchers narrowed down to precise questions about the extent to which the fundholding scheme promoted efficiency and preserved equity. They used one qualitative method, semistructured interviews, with the general practitioners and practice managers and also with people responsible for implementing the policy at national and regional level. The interviews were complemented by the collection of quantitative data such as financial information from the practices (box 1).

The second approach is more open and in effect starts by asking broad questions such as what is happening here? and, what are the important features and relationships that explain the impact of their intervention? These questions are then refined and become more specific in the course of fieldwork and a parallel process of data analysis. This type of design, in which the eventual research questions emerge during the research, is termed ethnography and has been advocated for use in the study of the impact of

---

Box 1—Outline of case study of GP fundholding[13]

- Mix of qualitative and quantitative methods
- Fundholding and non-fundholding practices
- Programme of interviews with key staff at practices
- Interviews with people responsible for implementing national policy
- Study found that the general practitioner fundholding scheme was achieving the aims set for it by government and that adverse selection ("cream skimming") of patients was less likely than some commentators had feared

---

government policies in the health system.[14 15] In some ways it is similar to the way in which consultations are conducted in that it involves initial exploration, progressing over time towards a diagnosis inferred from the available data.

The evaluation of resource management in the NHS,[16] which investigated the progress of six pilot hospitals in implementing new management arrangements, focused particularly on identifying ways in which doctors and general managers could jointly control the allocation and commitment of resources (box 2). At the outset the nature of resource management was unclear—sites were charged with finding ways of involving doctors in management, but how this would be achieved and, if achieved, how successful it would be in improving patient care were open questions. The researchers selected major specialties within each site and con-

---

Box 2—Evaluation of resource management[16]

- Six hospitals, a mix of teaching and non-teaching
- Focus on major specialties: general surgery and general medicine
- Mix of qualitative and quantitative methods
- Methods and data sources independent of each other
- Qualitative methods included interviews, non-participant observation of meetings, analysis of documentation
- Evaluation found that there were important changes in management processes, but little evidence of improvement in patient care

---

ducted interviews with relevant staff, observed meetings, and analysed documentation. Over time, the data were used to develop a framework which captured the essential features of resource management at the time and which was used to evaluate each site's progress in implementing it.

Selection of sites

The process of selecting sites for study is central to the case study approach. Researchers have developed a number of selection strategies, the objectives of which, as in any good research study, are to ensure that misinterpretation of results is as far as possible avoided. Criteria include the selection of cases that are typical of the phenomenon being investigated, those in which a specific theory can be tested, or those that will confirm or refute a hypothesis.

Researchers will benefit from expert advice from those with knowledge of the subject being investigated, and they can usefully build into the initial research design the possibility of testing findings at further sites. Replication of results across sites helps to ensure that findings are not due to characteristics of particular sites; hence it increases external validity.[17]

Selection of methods

The next step is to select research methods, the process being driven by criteria of validity and reliability.[18] A distinctive but not unique feature of case study research is the use of multiple methods and sources of evidence to establish construct validity. The use of particular methods is discussed elsewhere in the book; the validity and reliability of individual methods is discussed in more detail in Chapter 2.

Case studies often use triangulation[20] to ensure the validity of findings. In triangulation all data items are corroborated from at least one other source and normally by another method of data collection. The fundholding study referred to earlier[13] used interviews in combination with several different quantitative sources of data to establish an overall picture. The evaluation of resource management, in contrast, used a wider range of qualitative and quantitative methods.[16]

Any one of these methods by itself might have produced results of weak validity, but the different methods were used to obtain data from different sources. When they all suggested the emergence of an important development, therefore, they acted to strengthen the researchers' belief in the validity of their observations.

Another technique is to construct chains of evidence; these are conceptual arguments that link phenomena to one another in the following manner: "if this occurs then some other thing would be expected to occur; and if not, then it would not be expected." For example, if quantitative evidence suggested that there had been an increase or decrease in admission rates in several specialties within a resource management site and if an interview programme revealed that the involvement of doctors in management (if developed as part of the resource management initiative) had led to a higher level of coordination of admissions policies, then this is evidence that resource management may facilitate the introduction of such policies. This type of argument is not always appropriate, but it can be valuable where it is important to investigate causation in complex environments.

Analytical frameworks

The collection of data should be directed towards the development of an analytical framework that will facilitate interpretation of findings. Again, there are several ways in which this might be done. In the study of fundholding[13] the data were organised to "test" hypotheses which were derived from pre-existing economic theories. In the cases of resource management there was no obvious pre-existing theory that could be used; the development of a framework during the study was crucial to help organise and evaluate the data collected. The framework was not imposed on the data but derived from it in an iterative process over the course of the evaluation; each was used to refine the other over time (box 3).[15]

The investigator is finally left with the difficult task of making a judgment about the findings of a study. The purpose of the steps in designing and building the case study research is to maximise confidence in the findings, but interpretation inevitably involves value judgments. The findings may well include divergences of opinion among those involved about the value of the intervention, and the results will often point towards different conclusions.

The extent to which research findings can be assembled into a single coherent account of events varies widely. In some circumstances widely differing opinions are themselves very important and should be reflected in any report. Where an evaluation is

---

Box 3—Framework: five interrelated elements of resource management[16]

- Commitment to resource management by the relevant personnel at each level in the organisation

- Devolution of authority for the management of resources

- Collaboration within and between disciplines in securing the objectives of resource management

- Management infrastructure, particularly in terms of organisational structure and provision of information

- A clear focus for the local resource management strategy

---

designed to inform policy making, however, some attempt has to be made at an overall judgment of success or failure; this was the case in the evaluation of resource management, where it was important to indicate to policy makers and the NHS whether it was worthwhile.

Conclusion

The complexity of the issues that health professionals have to deal with and the increasing recognition by policy makers, academics, and practitioners of the value of case studies in evaluating health service interventions suggest that the use of such studies is likely to increase in the future. Qualitative methods can be used within case study designs to address many practical and policy questions that impinge on the lives of professionals, particularly where those questions are concerned with how or why events take a particular course.

Further reading

Smith G, Cantley C. *Assessing health care: a study in organisational evaluation.* Milton Keynes: Open University Press, 1985.

Yin R. *Case study research: design and methods.* 2nd ed. Newbury Park, CA: Sage, 1994.

1 Robinson R. Hospitals in the market. In: Keen J, ed. *Information management in health services.* Milton Keynes: Open University Press, 1994:3–15.
2 Knapp M, Hardy B, Wistow G, Forder J. *Markets for social care: opportunities, barriers and implications.* Canterbury: University of Kent at Canterbury, 1993. (PSSRU discussion paper 919.)

3 Committee of Public Accounts. *Wessex Regional Health Authority regional information systems plan*. London: HMSO, 1993. (PAC 63rd report, House of Commons, Session 1992/93.)

4 Audit Commission. *A short cut to better services*. London: HMSO, 1990.

5 Office of Technology Assessment. *Unconventional cancer treatments*. Washington, DC: OTA, 1990. (Report H-405.)

6 National Audit Office. *National Health Service: hospital catering in England*. London: HMSO, 1994. (Report No 329.)

7 Pollitt C, Harrison S, Hunter D, Marnoch G. The reluctant managers: clinicians and budgets in the NHS. *Financial Accountability and Management* 1988;4:213–33.

8 Griffiths R. *NHS management inquiry*. London: DHSS, 1983. (Griffiths report.)

9 Secretaries of State. *Working for patients*. London: HMSO, 1989. (Cmnd 555.)

10 Robinson R, Le Grand J, eds. *Evaluating the NHS reforms*. London: King's Fund Institute, 1994.

11 Berwick D, Godfrey AB, Roessner J. *Curing health care*. San Francisco: Jossey Bass, 1991.

12 St Leger A, Schneider H, Walsworth-Bell J. *Evaluating health service effectiveness*. Milton Keynes: Open University Press, 1992.

13 Glennerster H. Matsaganis M, Owens P. *Implementing GP fundholding*. Milton Keynes: Open University Press, 1994.

14 Pollitt C, Harrison S, Hunter D, Marnoch G. No hiding place: on the discomforts of researching the contemporary policy process. *Journal of Social Policy* 1990;19:169–90.

15 Mays N, Pope C. Observational methods in health care settings. *BMJ* 1995;311:182–4.

16 Packwood T, Keen J, Buxton M. *Hospitals in transition: the resource management experiment*. Milton Keynes: Open University Press, 1991.

17 Patton M. *Qualitative evaluation and research methods*. 2nd ed. Newbury Park, CA: Sage, 1990.

18 Yin R. *Case study research: design and methods*. 2nd ed. Newbury Park, CA: Sage, 1994.

19 Mays N, Pope C. Rigour and qualitative research. *BMJ* 1995;311:109–12.

20 Jick T. Mixing qualitative and quantitative methods: triangulation in action. *Administrative Sciences Quarterly* 1979;24:602–11.

67

Appendix

Opening the black box: an encounter in the
corridors of health services research

CATHERINE POPE, NICHOLAS MAYS

BMJ 30 January 1993

**Health services research has become more prominent as a
result of the NHS reforms. Both providers and purchasers
want to know exactly where the money is spent and how it
could be used more effectively. How best to obtain information about health services is the subject of some debate
within and between disciplines engaged in such research.
Because of their training doctors are often sceptical of
anything other than formal clinical trials and research
which produces statistical data. Some sociologists argue
that another way to find out what is actually happening in
the NHS is to observe people at work and talk to them. This
article debates these different views of research methods.
For effective research both quantitative and qualitative
approaches need to be used.**

This paper presents a dialogue between two conflicting voices
from health services research. It is presented primarily to inform
and stimulate debate and it therefore adopts a style which is
unusual in this journal. The polarisation of views, inherent in the
structure of a dialogue, may oversimplify complex issues at the
heart of the debate, but we hope that it highlights several important
conflicts which remain unresolved.

The setting for the dialogue is the corridor outside the office of
the director of a large and successful health services research unit.
The director (who has an impressive record of quantitative

research) meets a recently appointed sociologist . . .

SOCIOLOGIST: I'm glad I've caught you. It's about this research proposal you've just turned down—what do you mean, "It's not proper health services research?"

DIRECTOR: Well, you were going to look at only two hospitals. What sort of a sample is that? Why don't you take up my earlier suggestion of doing a randomised controlled trial?

SOC: Because it won't tell you what you need to know. My project was a reasonable attempt to find out what's really going on in those two hospitals.

DIR: I'm sorry, but we have to convince the medical research establishment that we can deliver high quality work, not these small scale, unquantifiable studies of yours. Clinicians often see health services research as the soft option and easy to carry out. We need to win their respect.

SOC: And how, exactly, are you going to do that?

DIR: We've got to undertake good, credible, scientific research. Science is respected and understood by clinicians (after all, it's the foundation of medicine).

SOC: Do you mean science in general or a particular image of "hard" science like economics with all its equations? To my mind, what I do as a medical sociologist is just as scientific.

DIR: You're entitled to your view, naturally, but clinicians won't understand what you do. The model of science they know is an experimental one—the randomised controlled trial used to test drugs and surgical procedures. We can test health services in exactly the same way. A fraction of current health services research in the United Kingdom consists of randomised trials[1]; we need many more—you know the sort of thing, classic trials like Mather's work in the late 1960s[2,3] which compared the treatment of myocardial infarction at home and in the hospital coronary care unit. There was a higher mortality after a month in the group treated in hospital. A year later there was still a significant advantage for the patients who went home.

SOC: Hang on a minute. Wasn't that the trial where only about a quarter of the patients were actually randomised? It's hardly a celebration of the experimental method. It was fraught with problems.

DIR: Yes, but the study was repeated by another team. The second time the researchers randomised most of the patients and they showed no significant difference in mortality in the home and hospital groups at six weeks.[4] From these studies we've developed criteria to identify who needs to go to a coronary care unit and who doesn't.

Who applies the results of trials?

SOC: But does anyone actually use those criteria?

DIR: I don't know. I'm just a researcher—not a cardiologist. It's not my job to implement research. All I do is produce basic knowledge.

SOC: As far as I can see, your contribution to basic knowledge is well and truly ignored. Not just in coronary care—there are other examples. Numerous trials have evaluated the various procedures performed during pregnancy and labour (Iain Chalmers has even gone to the trouble of collating them) but very few of these ideas have changed obstetric practice.[5]

DIR: I can't help it if some clinicians are cussed. Anyway, you can't dismiss the experimental method just because some irrational people choose not to put the findings into practice. Randomised trials have enormous potential for improving health policy—at a much higher level than individual specialties like coronary care or obstetrics. Take something as fundamental as the NHS and Community Care Act[6]—we could have tested whether general practitioner fundholding was better than health care purchasing by districts. We should have done something like the RAND health insurance experiment.[7][8]

SOC: The what?

DIR: The huge project in the United States which randomised people to different health insurance schemes to look at the consequences, including the impact on their health. That's the kind of work we should be getting into here.

SOC: I'm sorry, but I still have real problems with this picture of the experiment as an ideal. This is a modern health services research unit but you hold an antiquated view of science. It only seems to include the experimental model drawn from the natural sciences. I'm not even convinced that the natural sciences actually work like that[9] and I'm not sure you have any right to assert that the randomised controlled trial is the best method. It has its limitations.

Alternatives to experiments

DIR: I think you're just against experiments.

SOC: Not entirely, but your "one best method" argument reminds me of a very old debate in sociology about positivism . . .

DIR: Do you have to talk in "isms"? If you could put it in plain English I must be able to understand.

SOC: Let me draw an analogy, then. The different methods employed by social scientists are like the different views of the surgeon and the epidemiologist. Surgeons learn through direct experience of individual cases—through what they see, hear, and feel at their fingertips. In contrast the epidemiologist views the surgeon's patients at the aggregate level as clusters of variables. Have you got that?

DIR: Yes, but I've never given much credence to anecdotal evidence from surgeons. Go on.

SOC: Well, between these two extremes there is a whole range of theoretical perspectives and research methods to choose from, both qualitative and quantitative. What I want, returning to my analogy, is for the surgeon's view to be given a place in the scheme of research alongside the epidemiologist's. Methodological pluralism is vital in an applied subject like health services research. Even the Medical Research Council recognises that health services research "is typically multidisciplinary, bringing together as appropriate expertise in biological and clinical science, epidemiology, statistics, economics and the social sciences."[10] If you only use experiments you're using a very limited tool box.

DIR: I wasn't arguing just for randomised controlled trials—but we do need hard facts like those which experiments provide.

SOC: Yes, but you judge all facts using hard science as your gold standard. The point is that some things in health services can't easily be looked at with quantitative methods alone. Qualitative methods could help by looking at health care organisation and delivery—at the processes of care.

What is meant by process?

DIR: But process is simply what health services do to patients. We're interested in the product of health care, the outcome, the results of intervention.[11] If the patient dies it's a bad outcome and I know there's something wrong with the process. End of story.

SOC: That's oversimplifying the situation. We need a wider definition of process. It's more than just what happens to individual patients. It's also about organisations and the people within them— not just the patient who dies, but the doctors, nurses, auxiliaries, planners, administrators, clerks, and porters, and the noisy, chaotic interaction between them and the structure that surrounds them. There is a black box marked process and we haven't even begun to open it.

DIR: So what exactly would you do?

SOC: Well, for a start, I would open up our full methodological tool box and start using techniques other than randomised trials and models of research borrowed from epidemiology. Perhaps health services researchers could begin to use some of the qualitative techniques available.

DIR: Aha! I knew it. You want us to conform to your orthodoxy. . .

SOC: No, mine isn't the only approach. All I'm asking is that you begin to take these methods seriously and consider them alongside your own quantitative skills. After all, market researchers in the no nonsense world of retailing and commerce often use qualitative and quantitative methods together.

DIR: What exactly are these qualitative methods you're offering?

SOC: Well, what about observational studies, for a start?

DIR: But we do lots of those. We've done lots of comparative work, case-control studies . . .

SOC: Oh dear! We're not even talking the same language here. I didn't mean case-control studies. I meant observation. You know, being there, looking, and listening. I was thinking of ethnography, which means you have to immerse yourself in the situation and talk to the people involved like an anthropologist would.[12] That's just one example of an approach which gets away from counting events and controlling for extraneous variables. It's about trying to understand what is going on, almost through the eyes of the participants themselves.

DIR: Sounds like an excuse to loaf around doing nothing in particular to me. What can ethnography tell us about the big issues? For instance, I bet it can't help us solve the problem of waiting lists? Can your precious ethnography tell us anything which would be of practical use about managing these queues?

Value of ethnography

SOC: Only that they're not queues. Isn't that worth knowing?

DIR: What pretentious, counterintuitive rubbish. We might not know how best to manage waiting lists, but we don't need sociologists to complicate the basics by telling us they're not queues. They're great long queues of people waiting to go into hospital.

SOC: No, they're not. By saying they're like bus queues, you've made lots of assumptions. If you really want to understand a waiting list you need to get in there and find out how it is organised and managed. The best way of doing this is to study the people who actively assemble and maintain the waiting lists. Then you see that waiting lists seldom resemble anything like the formal queue which operations researchers are so fond of modelling.

DIR: I'm still puzzled about how you got this idea.

SOC: By studying one district in detail using the ethnographic methods I described.[13] By observing how a list is managed I found out that although lists are kept chronologically, patients seldom come off the list in that order. The office staff and the surgeons used the list as a pool of work they would dip into—indeed a surgeon might deliberately choose a recent addition to the list over someone who had waited far longer on the grounds of greater urgency . . .

DIR: And quite right too.

SOC: . . . or simply because they remembered the patient. There were all sorts of other processes that worked against the idea of a simple queue which managers needed to know about.

DIR: I take your point, but what about wider, international debates? What about explaining variations in the rates of common surgical procedures like cholecystectomy and hysterectomy between regions and countries. Quantitative work by people like McPherson, Wennberg, and so on[14] can tell us about that variation.

SOC: And I suppose you'd like more of the same so you can go on pinpointing variation and replicate the studies which have been done to show the same thing in different places, or maybe to include a few more explanatory variables in your statistical model?

DIR: Well, yes . . .

SOC: But clinical variation raises other questions which need to be answered. What we really need to do now is start uncovering how those rates are generated by the actions of individual clinicians.

Take something like Wennberg's concept of the surgical signature, used to describe the different profile of surgical work performed by different surgeons.[15] What we need to know is how those "signatures" get written. And this gets us back to looking at process. We need to know the sequence of events which take place before the patterns of surgical variation are produced.

DIR: So what do you think your approach can offer?

SOC: For one thing, it could tell us more about how variation is constructed. Mick Bloor's qualitative work on adenotonsillectomy is a perfect example of the kind of study I'm talking about.[16] He carried out an observational study of ear, nose, and throat outpatient clinics and showed that there were systematic variations in patient assessment routines among consultants, rooted in differences between the specialists in their informal decision making rules. If you combine such work with quantitative data you can begin to explain how variation occurs.

Outsider's view of sociology

DIR: Your programme for looking at process is all very well, but this is exactly what your lot, medical sociologists, have ignored.[17] Medical sociology has long since given up looking at process—it's too busy experiencing illness and waffling on about doctor-patient interaction.

SOC: Perhaps, but part of the reason lies in the culture of health services research. In the United Kingdom it's driven by medicine and there aren't many posts for social scientists.[18] You only have to look at what gets funded and who evaluates the proposals. There's very little room for the qualitative work I've been talking about: if it is there it tends to get tacked on to an existing project when the sociologist is brought in to provide expertise on survey design or interviewing or to use a standard measure of patient "quality of life."

DIR: You can't blame me for your failure to secure funding. Anyway isn't the Medical Research Council canvassing medical sociologists for grant applications?[19]

SOC: Yes, but they mostly seem to have people like you assessing the proposals. It's no good having people who know nothing about qualitative research applying their yardsticks of experimental science to all types of research.

DIR: Well then, I certainly can't argue your case for you. I only know about my approach.

SOC: But you could back my project?

DIR: The decision's made. But I'll tell you what we'll do. Come back to me in a few weeks with another research proposal. After today's discussion I should be a bit better at understanding what you're driving at!

SOC: That's something, I suppose.

DIR: Could I make one last suggestion? Your research proposal wasn't very user friendly. You could do worse than take a leaf out of the health economists' book. When I started out, nobody had heard of health economics; now every provider unit in the health service wants one. People seem to want health economists, up to a point, and even epidemiologists because they boast a set of tools to offer managers and doctors for opening what you called the black box. The economists didn't get to this position by hanging back and whingeing from the sidelines. If, as you claim, medical sociology, and your ethnographic methods, can really open up this realm, of process and tell us what is going on in the "black box" then you've got to be more entrepreneurial. Change your name to Pandora while you're at it; people might be less inclined to be dismissive!

1 Fowkes FRG, Garraway WM, Sheehy CK. The quality of health services research in medical practice in the United Kingdom. *BMJ* 1991;45:102–6.
2 Mather HG, Pearson NG, Read KLQ, Shaw DB, Steed GR, Morgan DC, et al. Myocardial infarction: home and hospital treatment. *BMJ* 1971;iii. 334–8.
3 Mather HG, Morgan DC, Pearson NG, Read KLQ, Shaw DB, Steed GR, et al. Acute Myocardial infarction: a comparison between home and hospital care for patients. *BMJ* 1976;i:925–9.
4 Hill JD, Hampton JR, Mitchell JRA. A randomised trial of home versus hospital management for patients with suspected myocardial infarction. *Lancet* 1978;i:837–41.
5 Chalmers I, Enkin M, Keise MJNC. *Effective care in pregnancy and childbirth*. Oxford: Oxford University Press, 1989.
6 *National Health Service and Community Care Act 1990*. London: HMSO, 1990.
7 Ware JE, Brook RH, Rogers WH, Keeler EB, Davis AR, Sherbourne CD et al. Comparison of health outcomes at a health maintenance organisation with those of fee-for-service care. *Lancet* 1986;i:1017–22.
8 Welch BL, Hay JW, Miller DS, Olsen RJ, Rippey RM, Welch AS. The Rand health insurance study: a summary critique. *Med Care* 1987;25:148–56.
9 Bhasker R. *The possibility of naturalism: a philosophical critique of the contemporary human sciences*. Sussex: Harvester Press, 1979.
10 Medical Research Council. *Corporate strategy, 1989*. London: MRC, 1989:48.
11 Cochrane AL. *Effectiveness and efficiency: random reflections on health services*. London: Nuffield Provincial Hospitals Trust, 1972.
12 Hammersley M, Atkinson P. *Ethnography: principles in practice*. London: Tavistock, 1983.
13 Pope C. Trouble in store: some thoughts on the management of waiting lists. *Sociology of Health and Illness* 1993;13:193–212.
14 McPherson K, Wennberg JE, Hovind O, Clifford P. Small area variations in the use of common surgical procedures: an international comparison of New England, England and Norway. *N Engl J Med* 1982;307:1310–4.
15 Wennberg J, Gittelsohn A. Variations in medical care among small areas. *Scientific American* 1982;246:100–11.

16 Bloor M, Bishop Berkeley and the adenotonsillectomy enigma: an exploration of variation in the social construction of medical disposals. *Sociology* 1976;**10**:43–61.

17 Hunter D. Organizing and managing health care: a challenge for medical sociology. In: Cunningham-Burley S, McKeganey NP, eds. *Readings in medical sociology.* London: Tavistock/Routledge, 1990: 213–36.

18 Clarke M, Kurinczuk JJ, for Committee of Heads of Academic Departments of Public Health Medicine. Health services research: a case of need or special pleading? *BMJ* 1992;**304**:1675–6.

19 Peatfield AC. The Medical Research Council, health services research and social science. *Medical Sociology News* 1992;**17**(2):15.

Index

Also from the BMJ Publishing Group

SYSTEMATIC REVIEWS
Edited by Iain Chalmers, Doug Altman

With over two million health research papers published each year, systematic reviews are needed to provide manageable information on which decisions on health policy, and individual treatment, can be based. In this book the leading authorities in this subject illustrate how traditional reviews sometimes arrive at lethally incorrect conclusions and show how the quality of reviews can be improved. They describe how to prepare a good review and how to evaluate one.
ISBN 0 7279 0904 5

HOW TO WRITE A PAPER
Edited by G M Hall

This short book provides all the practical information on how to get a paper accepted. It has chapters on each section of a scientific paper from Introduction to Discussion. With contributions from editors of international journals including the *BMJ*, *British Journal of Anaesthesia*, and *Cardiovascular Research*, it explains in a refreshingly direct way what journal editors are looking for in a good paper.
ISBN 0 7279 0822 7

OUTCOMES INTO CLINICAL PRACTICE
Edited by Tony Delamothe

Outcomes research, the new buzz word in health care, refers to the generation, collection, and analysis of the results of medical care. Such information offers the opportunities to improve clinical effectiveness and set standards for good practice. Based on a ground breaking conference held by the *BMJ, BMA,* and UK Clearing House, *Outcomes into Clinical Practice* discusses the issues involved and gives real examples of how outcomes research works best.

ISBN 0 7279 0888 X

For further details contact your local bookseller, or in case of difficulty, contact the Books Division, BMJ Publishing Group, BMA House, Tavistock Square, London WC1H 9JR, UK (Tel +44(0) 171-383-6245; Fax +44(0) 171-383 6662)